ISOMETRIC EXERCISE AND ITS CLINICAL IMPLICATIONS

ISOMETRIC EXERCISE AND ITS CLINICAL IMPLICATIONS

By

JERROLD SCOTT PETROFSKY, Ph.D.

Biomedical Engineering Laboratory
Departments of Engineering and Physiology
Wright State University
Dayton, Ohio

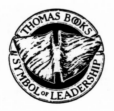

CHARLES C THOMAS • PUBLISHER
Springfield • Illinois • U.S.A.

QP
301
P397

Published and Distributed Throughout the World by
CHARLES C THOMAS• PUBLISHER
2600 South First Street, Springfield, Illinois, U.S.A., 62717

©*1982, by* CHARLES C THOMAS• PUBLISHER
ISBN 0-398-04520-8
Library of Congress Catalog Card Number: 81-5294

*With THOMAS BOOKS Careful attention is given to all details of manufacturing and
design. It is the Publisher's desire to present books that are satisfactory as to their physical
qualities and artistic possibilities and appropriate for their particular use. THOMAS
BOOKS will be true to those laws of quality that assure a good name and good will.*

Library of Congress Cataloging in Publication Data

Petrofsky, Jerrold Scott.
 Isometric exercise and its clinical implications.

 Bibliography: p.
 Includes index.
 1. Isometric exercise — Physiological aspects.
I. Title. [DNLM: 1. Exertion. WE 103 P497i]
QP301.P397   613.7'1   81-5294
ISBN 0-398-04520-8   AACR2

Printed in the United States of America
AF-R-1

This book is dedicated to my wife, Cheryl,
my daughter, Missy, and
Professor Alexander R. Lind
for introducing me to this area.

We shall not cease from exploration
And at the end of our exploring
Will be to arrive where we started
And know the place for the first time.

"Little Gidding," V
—T.S. Eliot

PREFACE

The contraction of skeletal muscle can be subdivided into two categories: static contractions and dynamic contractions. Static exercise involves contractions where the muscle does not change length. Isometric exercise differs from dynamic exercise in many ways. The most dramatic of these is perhaps the blood pressure response. It was this response that originally sparked interest in the area due to the early work of Asmusson (1938) and Alam and Smirk (1937, 1938A, 1938B). These early investigators in the area found that unlike most types of dynamic exercise where the mean blood pressure even during maximal work usually does not increase above resting values, the blood pressure during fatiguing isometric exercise increases sharply above that at rest. For example, during a contraction lasting about two minutes at a tension of 40 percent of the maximum strength of the handgrip muscles (MVC), in our own work (Petrofsky and Lind 1975A) we found that the average individual will have an increase of about 50 percent above resting values in the systolic, diastolic, and mean blood pressures. However, the range of response is large. In some individuals the blood pressure response is modest, whereas in others the blood pressure can more than double during a two-minute isometric contraction.

Much of the early work concerning isometric exercise was centered around this dramatic blood pressure response that occurs during this form of effort. But after the initial interest in the area in the 1930s not much happened for the next twenty years. Interest in the pressure response was rekindled by the classic studies by Lind and his colleagues (1959, 1964). These studies examined the relationship between strength and endurance during isometric contractions. The specific relationship between strength and endurance during isometric exercise was finally

vii

published in the mid-1960s when Monod and Scherrer, and later Rohmert, presented what is now their classic curves relating strength and endurance for isometric contractions (Monod and Scherrer 1967; Rohmert 1968), often called the *Rohmert curve*.

The first complete description of the physiology of isometric exercise was published in a chapter by Simonson and Lind in the textbook of work physiology by Simonson in 1971. No complete description of the physiology of isometric exercise has been published since then. However, since the discovery of the neural pathways involved in the heart rate and blood pressure response to isometric exercise in the early 1970s, the literature on isometric exercise has increased exponentially, culminating with a recent international symposium on the cardiovascular responses to isometric exercise held in Dallas, Texas, in 1979 and a symposium on muscle fatigue during isometric contractions held at the twenty-eighth Congress of the International Physiology Society in Budapest in 1980.

In the last ten years the interest in isometric exercise and the associated physiological responses has taken several different directions. Because of the dramatic increase in afterload on the heart during fatiguing isometric exercise, the physiology of isometric exercise is still important to the clinician, since isometric exercise poses a potentially hazardous load on the cardiovascular system of a patient with a compromised myocardium or for the patient with an aneurysm.

Obviously, basic research into the relationship between strength and endurance and the cardiorespiratory response to isometric exercise has continued. Although isometric exercise is a fairly common type of exercise encountered often in everyday life, many types of dynamic exercise include isometric exercise as well, and as will be described later in this book, the physiological responses to combined static and dynamic exercise are additive. Further, there exists a static component of most types of dynamic exercise. Lifting weights slowly or lifting heavy boxes is a type of dynamic exercise with a very high static component. Here again, the cardiorespiratory responses during this form of exertion are much more pronounced than during pure dynamic exercise alone.

Recent advances in technology have once again increased interest in the field of isometric exercise physiology. With the explosion in aerospace technology that has occurred in the last fifteen to twenty years, man is now exposed to exotic environments. For example, in a spacecraft orbiting earth man is exposed to a zero G environment. Habituation in this environment is associated with marked cardiovascular deconditioning. To make matters worse, to move a lever with a hand in a zero G environment necessitates the other hand and both legs being placed in hand and foot holds and contracting isometrically to stabilize the body position. In contrast, in vectored wing fighter aircraft, man is now exposed to high G forces in both the $+G_z$ and $+G_y$ directions. Under these conditions, pilots exert intense isometric contractions during flight maneuvers. These maneuvers result in heavy isometric contractions not only to the arms and legs, but especially in the neck muscles, which must support an aircraft helmet weighted with heavy avionics packages.

This book will be divided into three parts. In the first part (Chapters 1, 2, 3 and 4) the physiology of isometric exercise and the blood pressure, heart rate, and ventilation responses during this form of exertion will be examined. In addition, motor unit recruitment patterns and the electromyogram (EMG) during isometric exercise will also be discussed. In a second section (Chapters 5 and 6), the electrical, metabolic and cardiorespiratory responses to isometric exercise will be used as a tool with which to examine potential mechanisms and locations for the muscle fatigue that occurs during isometric exercise. Finally, in the last section (Chapter 7), the clinical implications and use of isometric exercise will be explored. The book is written at a level that is both suitable for the graduate student and experienced researcher in the area.

J.S.P.

ACKNOWLEDGEMENTS

I wish to gratefully acknowledge the invaluable help of Miss Dawn Greenwell, Miss Karen Hopkins, Dr. Chandler Phillips, and Mr. Bruce Stiver in the preparation of this book.

CONTENTS

ISOMETRIC EXERCISE AND ITS CLINICAL IMPLICATIONS

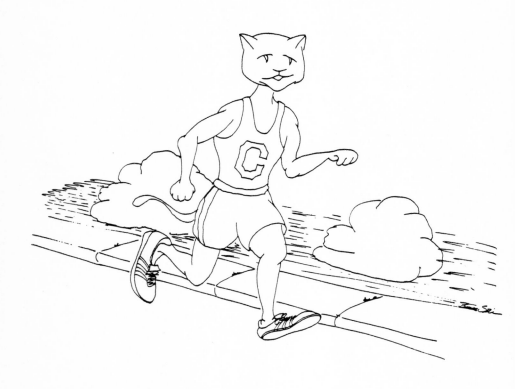

CHAPTER 1

ISOMETRIC TRAINING

ISOMETRIC STRENGTH TRAINING

T he effect of muscle activity or inactivity on the strength and endurance of muscle has been studied extensively in the past fifty years. Certainly, one long-held axiom in the exercise literature has been confirmed over and over: training for a particular task must involve training of the muscles, which are to accomplish the work, and the training must involve the type of work being trained for. Isometric training is not an effective means of training a muscle for dynamic exercise, and dynamic training has no influence on isometric performance (De Lorme and Watkins 1951; Astrand and Rodahl 1970; Hansen 1967; Petersén et al. 1961). For example, in a study by Petersen et al. (1961), the effect of dynamic and static training on dynamic and static performance was measured. Isometric training (60% maximal voluntary strength [MVC] @ 150 contractions per day) resulted in a marked increase in static performance but little effect on dynamic performance. With dynamic training the reverse was true (*See* Table 1-I). In contrast, a reduction in physical activity due to bed rest (Saltin et al. 1968; Greenleaf et al. 1977), immobilization in a cast (Gutmann 1976; Müller 1970; Stillwell 1967), or tenotomy (Vrobóva 1963) will reduce the strength of a muscle. During immobilization, fast-twitch motor units lose strength and gain oxidative capacity, taking on the appearance of slow-twitch motor units. This appears to be due to the influence of the motor nerve on the muscle (neurotrophic effect) (Gottman 1976), since cross innervation of fast- and slow-twitch muscle has a similar effect (Barany and Close 1971; Buller et al. 1960, 1971). When an extremity is immobilized in a cast, the loss in strength is greater than that which occurs during bed rest. Müller and Hettinger (1953) proposed that if subjects sustained brief contractions (a few seconds) at tensions greater than one-third of the maximum strength of the muscle each day, the reduction in strength (usually around 20%) would be eliminated. This early observation (which was confirmed by Rozier et al. 1979) formed a basis for much of the use of isometrics by weight lifters. It was assumed that a few isometric contractions each day would cause rapid increases in muscle strength. However, in our own experience, when subjects have exerted MVC's as many as 10 times per day, intermixed with fatiguing submaximal isometric contractions sustained as many as 5 times per day, we have never seen an increase of more than 10 percent in isometric strength (Petrofsky and Lind 1975, Petrofsky, Burse, and Lind 1975). This is also the case for weight lifters (Astrand and Rohahl 1970). Further, Zimkin (1960) found that in initial training of strength, small increases in strength could be achieved by performing contractions at greater than one-third of the maximum strength, but the load had to be continually increased day by day to continue increasing muscle strength. In light of these results, Müller and Rohmert (1963) and Hettinger (1968) have modified their position. One difference between these observations and those of Müller may lie in the type of isometric contractions that are performed. Typically, in our own experiments, subjects performed pure isometric contractions. Where studies have reported large increases in isometric strength, muscle contractions were typically isokinetic; that is, although high tensions were exerted, the muscle was allowed change length at a very slow rate. This type of isometric training falls somewhere between dynamic and static exercise, since, as described in a later chapter, this form of exercise has a high static component and probably provides the best means of causing a rapid increase in muscle strength. Electrical stimulation of muscle has been shown to have a beneficial effect in preventing the loss of strength during immobilization and in achieving increases in strength in athletes (Eriksson and Haggmark 1979; Pette et al. 1973, 1975).

One obvious benefit of isometric training is in training the individual to exert a maximal effort repeatedly. In well-trained

Training	Maximal strength		Endurance 60% of maximum		Study
	(1) Isometric, kp x cm*	(2) Dynamic, kp†	(3) Isometric No. of contractions	(4) Dynamic, kpm	
Dynamic "60%" 150 contr./day 30 days	378 to 400 +6%	8.8 to 11.4 +29%		16.4 to 843 +5040%	Petersen et al, 1961
Isometric "60%" 150 constr./day 30 days	425 to 441 +4%	10.7 to 11.3 +6%	29 to 336 +100%	17 to 24 +41%	Hansen, 1961
Dynamic "60%" 100 contr./hour		12.1 to 13.7 +13%	100 to 98 -2%	60 to 438 +630%	Hansen, 1967

*Torque.
†Weight was lifted 25 cm.

TABLE 1-I

Measurement before and after training of maximal strength, of the arm flexors in (1) isometric and (2) dynamic contractions. Endurance tested with load that was 60 percent of the maximal strength and number of contractions (kpm) counted before fatigue made further successful contractions impossible for (3) isometric and (4) dynamic exercise. Training restricted to one type of muscle work at a time. The figures give the average performance before (e.g., 378 kp x cm) and after (e.g., 400 kp x cm) training as well as the percentage difference from Petersen et al. (1961).

and highly motivated subjects repeated isometric strength measurements have a high repeatability.

Ikai and Steinhaus (1961), for example, found that the maximum strength of their subjects could be increased by 7–12 percent by simply shouting at the subject. Hypnosis, in some subjects, will also increase strength (Levitt and Brady 1964). The maximum strength has also been shown to be increased if subjects are given knowledge of their score in a strength test (Berger 1967; Johnson and Nelson 1967). These increases in strength occur in the absence of hypertrophy of the muscle (Bowers 1966; Coleman 1969; DeVries 1968; Hellebrandt et al. 1947; Moritani and DeVries 1979). However, if the dynamometer is accurate and subjects are highly motivated, isometric strength does not increase even under hypnosis (Barber 1966). In large groups of subjects, strength measurements are quite repeatable. Rohmert (1961) and Muller (1961) both showed that the coefficient of variation (standard deviation ÷ mean) of strength measurements was ±8.5 percent. Tornvall (1963) found that for different muscle groups, the coefficient of variation ranged from 3.2–11.4 percent. Certainly, much of this variation is due to the complexity (number of muscles involved) in the contractions. The more complex the movement, the higher the coefficient of variation in repeated strength measurements. A summary of the coefficient of variations of repeated strength measurements by various investigators is shown in Table 1-II.

TABLE 1-II

Repeatability of Endurance Measurements

Study	*Coefficient of Variation*
Rohmert (1961)	8.5%
Müller (1961)	8.5%
Tornvall (1963)	3.2 to 11.4%
Start and Graham (1964)	7.1%
Martens and Sharkey (1966)	11.1%
Bruce et al (1968)	4.5%
Elbel (1949)	3-8%

ISOMETRIC ENDURANCE TRAINING

When fatiguing isometric contractions are sustained as many as ten times per day, we have not been able to detect any increases in isometric endurance. However, the coefficient of variation of endurance is typically reduced over a period of 4–6 weeks to less than 3 percent in a well-trained and highly motivated subject from day to day. Typically, in our own isometric endurance studies, we train subjects for 4–6 weeks by having them exert a series of 5 fatiguing isometric contractions each day; 3 minutes are allowed in between the contractions. We have found this is an acceptable training regimen for all studies, and in well-motivated subjects, the coefficient of variation in endurance from day to day is generally around 5 percent. In general, the repeatability of endurance measurements is not as good as that of strength, although Start and Graham (1964) found the correlation coefficient for repeated strength measurements to be 0.94; for endurance measurements it was only 0.83. Martens and Sharkey (1966) found the coefficient of variation in strength to be 11.1 percent, whereas for endurance it was 18.1 percent.

However, many factors such as muscle temperature can alter isometric endurance.

Hanson et al. (1967) and Petersen et al. (1961) found that dynamic training of short duration has no effect on endurance for isometric exercise. This has been confirmed with other types of light dynamic training. But, the biochemical makeup of muscle can be changed by physical training. It has been well established in the literature that heavy training for long periods of time with endurance types of exercise will result in the muscle changing biochemically toward the appearance of slow-twitch muscle (Holloszy and Booth 1976; Gollnick and King 1969; Gollnick et al. 1967, 1972; Barnard and Peter 1969; Barnard et al. 1970; Fitts et al. 1973, 1975). In contrast, isokinetic types of training usually result in muscle appearing biochemically as if it was predominately fast-twitch muscle. Therefore, it is not surprising that Astrand and Rodahl (1970) found that people who continually sustained isometric tensions day after day, such as professional motorcycle riders, had greater isometric endurance than in control groups. The exact relationship between fiber composition and endurance in man has yet to be explored.

The Effect of Isometric Training on the Cardiovascular System

Unlike dynamic exercise where marked cardiovascular conditioning takes place during training, there is little if any effect of isometric training on the heart. Both rhythmic (Rohter et al. 1963) and static (Vanderhoof et al. 1961) training have been shown to have little effect on resting or postexercise blood flows. However, isometric training of the handgrip muscles can increase both endurance and exercise blood flows (Byrd and Hills 1972). Since isokinetic strength training can result in hypertrophy of the muscle fibers (DeLorme and Watkins 1951; Hettinger and Müller 1953), the muscle mass is larger, but no evidence has been shown to prove that there is an increase in capillary density in this form of training. However, Komi et al. (1978) did find that isometric training increased enzyme activities of MDH, SDH, and HK, while lowering the activities of LDH and CPK, thereby improving efficiency of contraction at submaximal loads and enhancing the oxidative capacity of the muscle.

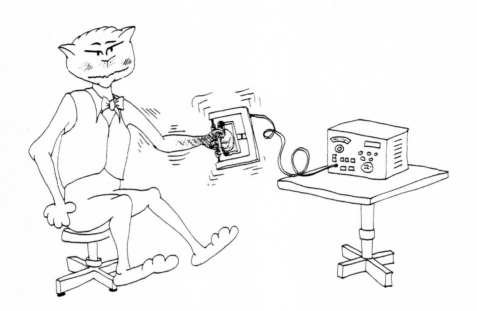

CHAPTER 2

ISOMETRIC STRENGTH AND ENDURANCE

ISOMETRIC STRENGTH

Although isometric strength varies greatly between individuals, the average isometric strength is generally about 30 percent greater in men than women (Petrofsky and Lind 1975A; Cotton and Bonnell 1969; Kearny et al. 1976; Kroll 1971; Wilmore 1974). The average isometric strength of the handgrip muscles in a recent study, for example, (Petrofsky and Lind 1975) was 49.2 kilograms in men and 28.9 kilograms in women. A number of factors can affect isometric strength. From birth, strength continually increases until the age of about thirty years — an age when most people have their greatest isometric strength (Larsson and Karlsson 1978; Larsson et al. 1979; Murray et al. 1980). From this age there is a gradual decline in strength throughout life as shown in Figure 2-1 for both men and women. Although the rate of decline in strength with age can be reduced by physical training (Astrand and Rodahl 1970), this decline still occurs in all individuals. A loss of motor units within the muscle is due to the destruction of alpha motorneurons within the central nervous system (Guttman and Hanzlekova 1972).

Muscle Temperature

Muscle temperature will also alter isometric strength. Most muscles in the body are located in shell tissues. Therefore, unlike the core tissues whose temperatures are regulated around 37° C, the temperature of shell tissues is not closely regulated. In warm weather, the blood flow is increased through shell tissues to allow the body to achieve greater heat exchange with the environment. In contrast, in cold weather, when heat in the body is conserved,

9

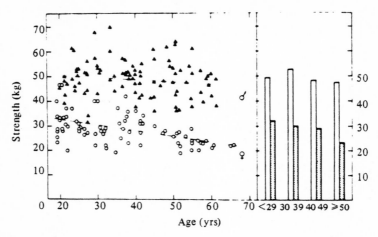

Figure 2-1.   The left panel represents the individual handgrip strengths of
each of the 100 men (▲) and 83 women (○) of different ages. Regression lines are drawn for each sex. Bar graphs in the right-
hand panel display the average strength for each decade for men
(hollow bars) and women (hatched bars). From Petrofsky and
Lind, Aging, Isometric Strength and Endurance, and the Cardiovascular Responses to Static Effort, *J Appl Physiol, 38*:91–95,
1975. Courtesy of The American Physiological Society.

blood flow is reduced, and the temperature of shell tissues approaches that of the environment. Therefore, it is not uncom-
mon to see variations in the temperature of, for example, the
forearm muscles by as much as 20° C between very cold and very
warm environments (Barcroft and Millen 1939; Clarke, Hellon,
and Lind 1958; Petrofsky and Lind 1975). Over the range of
muscle temperatures of 28° to 38° C, the maximum isometric
strength that can be developed by muscles (MVC) varies very little. However, when the muscle temperature is reduced below
28° C, strength declines rapidly as shown for the handgrip muscles for human subjects in Figure 2-2 (Clarke, Hellon, and Lind
1958). Part of this decline has been attributed to failure of contractile components in the muscle, but part of the decline in
strength also appears to be due to cold-related neuromuscular
junction failure (Cullingham et al. 1960; Petrofsky and Lind
1981).

Reliability

One problem that often plagues studies where isometric strength is measured is the reliability of strength measurements in any subject from day to day. Some studies have reported a wide variation in muscular strength from day to day in the same individual. Certainly, part of this problem is due to the dynamometer used to measure strength. A number of types of dynamometers are currently in use for strength measurements. Many of these dynamometers are spring-type dynamometers. Since the dynamometer must move a variable distance to distend the spring, these dynamometers are not true isometric dynamometers, and the reliability of repeated strength measurements is sometimes low. Part of this is due to the fact that the strength of the muscles of the body varies at different muscle lengths. For example, for the handgrip muscles there exists one handgrip size for gripping hand tools at which the muscles exert the maximum isometric strength for both men and women, as shown in Figure 2-3. As the hand is adjusted to narrower or wider dimensions, strength declines rapidly (Petrofsky et al. 1981). A more dramatic example would be the biceps muscles.

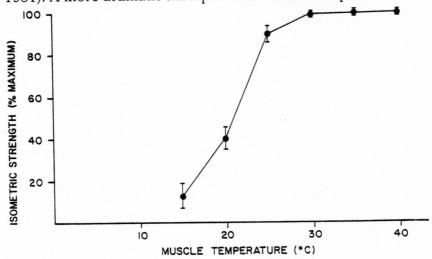

Figure 2-2.   The isometric strength of the handgrip muscles of 6 male subjects after immersion of their arms for 30 minutes in water between 5°–40° C to adjust their muscle temperature between 15°–40° C.

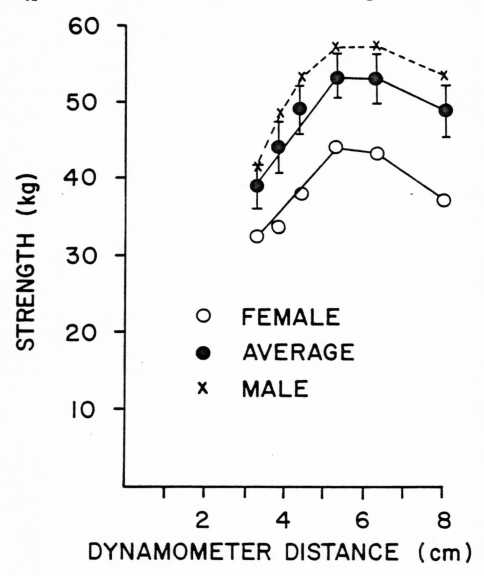

Figure 2-3.   This figure shows the average maximum voluntary strength of
the 8 male and 8 female subjects measured at differing grip
spans. Each mean is shown ± the respective standard deviations.
From Petrofsky et al., the Effect of Handgrip Span on Isometric
Performance, *Ergonomics*, 1981. Courtesy of Ergonomics.

For this muscle group, the angle of the elbow is quite critical in determining the maximum strength developed by the muscles; an elbow angle of approximately 120° is necessary for the muscles to develop their maximum isometric strength (Ismail and Ranatunga 1978; Petrofsky and Phillips 1981). This same relationship holds for most muscles in the body. It is therefore necessary that a dynamometer, which measures strength, must do so with as little displacement as possible so that the contractions are truly isometric.

Another problem that arises in strength measurements is assuring that the subject exerts his or her true MVC. In studies of human subjects, Ikai and Steinhaus (1961) found that the maximum voluntary strength of their subjects could be increased by shouting behind the subjects' back during the strength measurement. They therefore felt that most subjects did not truly exert a maximal effort in strength recordings. Due to differences in motivation from day to day, there would be a large variation in isometric strength. Further, in other studies with human subjects, it has been shown that electrical stimulation of skeletal muscle can cause the muscle to develop more strength than during the voluntary effort.

However, in a summary of some fifty studies involving hypnosis, Barber (1966) found that highly motivated human volunteers will exert the same isometric strength under hypnosis as is found during a voluntary effort. Merton also found that with highly motivated subjects, the maximum strength developed by the skeletal muscle could not be improved by electrical stimulation (1954). Therefore, it would appear that the critical factor in strength measurements is in using subjects who are highly motivated. With highly motivated subjects, the day to day coefficient of variation (standard deviation ÷ mean) in strength measurements is generally less than 5 percent (Tornvall 1963; Start and Graham 1964; Martens and Sharkey 1966; Elbel 1949; Donald et al. 1967).

ISOMETRIC ENDURANCE

Unlike dynamic exercise, the endurance for isometric exercise is quite short when the tension developed by the muscle exceeds 10–15 percent of the muscles maximum isometric strength.

Contractions below 10–15 percent MVC are said to be non-fatiguing because the tension can be held for an indefinite length of time with no apparent sign of muscle fatigue. However, as the tension developed by the muscle increases past 15 percent MVC, the length of time that the contraction can be sustained is reduced exponentially (Royce 1957; Monod and Scherrer 1967; Rohmert 1968; Petrofsky 1980C). For example, a contraction at a tension of 25 percent MVC can be typically sustained for a duration of about 8.5 minutes. In contrast, a contraction at 40 percent MVC can only be sustained for about 2.5 minutes, and a contraction at 70 percent MVC can only be sustained for about 30 seconds in most average subjects. The exact relationship between tension and isometric endurance was described first by Monod and Scherrer (1967) and later by Rohmert (1968) and is shown in Figure 2-4. Because of variations in strength between subjects, the X axis of a typical Rohmert curve is normalized in terms of the percent MVC sustained during the contractions. In

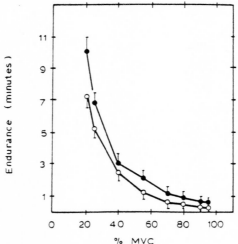

Figure 2-4.   The isometric endurance of the handgrip muscles in three female (●) and three male (○) subjects at tensions ranging between 20 and 95 percent MVC. Each point illustrates the mean of two determinations on each of the three subjects plus or minus the respective standard deviations. From Petrofsky, Computer Analysis of the Surface EMG During Isometric Exercise, *Comput Biol Med*, *10*:83–95, 1980. Courtesy of Computers in Biology and Medicine.

his original studies, Rohmert studied both male and female athletes, examining the strength endurance relationship in several different muscle groups. He concluded that endurance was the same in men and women and was unaffected by the size of the muscle group doing the exercise. However, the male and female subjects in his study were all of approximately the same age and same physical condition. Further, all experiments were conducted under exactly the same experimental conditions. It was not until some five years later that it was found that a large number of environmental and inherent factors can alter isometric endurance and that, in a normal population, endurance was different between women and men.

Temperature

As long as thirty years ago it was known that the temperature of the exercising muscle had a profound influence on isometric endurance. Hall, Mendoz, and Fitch (1947) showed that the application of hot packs above an exercising muscle would reduce isometric endurance. In contrast, cooling a muscle prior to isometric contraction increased isometric endurance. The exact relationship between temperature of the muscle and isometric endurance was first explored extensively by Clarke, Hellon, and Lind (1958) and confirmed later by Petrofsky and Lind (1975) and Edwards et al. (1972). In this classic study, Clarke, Hellon, and Lind found that there existed one muscle temperature at which a muscle could sustain isometric contractions the longest. In their experiments, contractions were sustained at one-third MVC to fatigue by male subjects. The results of their experiments can be summarized in Figure 2-5. The optimal temperature of the exercising muscle for sustaining a contraction at one-third MVC was 28° C; above and below this temperature isometric endurance decreased markedly. Over the muscle temperature range of 28°–38° C, the endurance will be reduced by about 66 percent if the muscle was warmed. The forearm muscle used in these experiments as an index of muscle temperature was the brachioradialis. These findings were particularly significant, because these investigators found the resting temperature of the brachioradialis muscle to be around 31°–32° C.

Since it has been shown that simply wearing a shirt or suitcoat can cause the muscle temperature of the brachioradialis to rise to 37° C, it would appear that the endurance for isometric contractions of the handgrip muscles could be potentially halved by wearing heavy clothing.

Body Fat

Factors other than environmental ones can alter isometric endurance as well. Body fat is a potent insulator found above

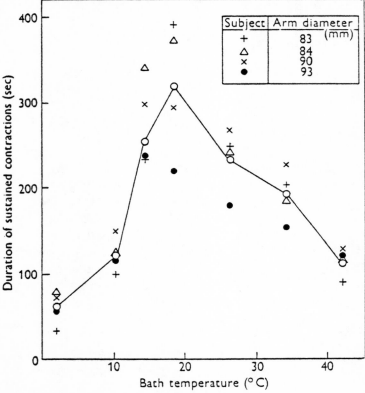

Figure 2-5.   Showing the individual (symbols) and mean (0–0) durations of the first five successive sustained contractions in water at seven temperatures. The diameter of the forearm of each subject, taken 6 cm above the mid position of the forearm, is shown inset. From Clarke, Hellon, and Lind, The Duration of Sustained Contractions of the Human Forearm, *J Physiol*, *143*:454–463, 1958. Courtesy of Journal of Physiology.

skeletal muscle in the body (Buskirk et al. 1963; Daniels and Baker 1961; Carlson et al. 1964; Keatinge and Evans 1960). Josenhans (1962) originally showed that overweight individuals had less endurance for a contraction at 100 percent MVC than normal weight subjects. Over 10 years later, in a population of 100 men and 83 women, Petrofsky and Lind (1975) found that there was an inverse relationship between body fat and isometric endurance for subjects sustaining fatiguing isometric contrac-

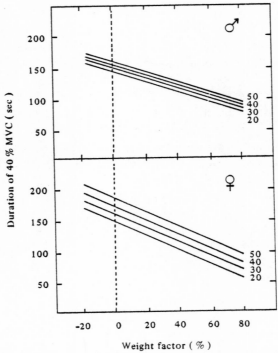

Figure 2-6. Multifactor analysis by multiple regression illustrates the relationship of isometric endurance (ordinate) to the weight factor (abscissa) and age (four curves for individuals of 20, 30, 40, and 50 years of age) in males (upper panel) and females (lower panel). The multiple regression equation for males is: y ($\pm$ 27.3) = 131.28 − 0.874 wt. + 0.534 age and for the females is: y ($\pm$ 48.8) = 1.429 age − 1.243 wt + 121.1. From Petrofsky and Lind, Isometric Strength Endurance, and the Blood Pressure and Heart Rate, *Europ J Physiol, 360*:49–61, 1975. Courtesy of Springer-Verlag New York, Inc.

tions of their handgrip muscles at a tension of 40 percent MVC. Body fat in these studies was estimated from the idealized height and weight charts established by the Metropolitan Life Insurance Company on 5 million people. From these ideal table values a weight factor was calculated as shown in the equation below:

$$\text{Wt factor} = \frac{\text{Wm-Wt}}{\text{Wt}} \; 100$$

where Wt = the ideal weight of the individual

Wm = the actual weight of the individual

If, for example, a person's weight was at the ideal weight for his height and sex, then the weight factor would be equal to zero. If a person was twice his ideal weight the weight factor would be 100 percent. Using this measure of body fat, a graph relating body fat to endurance was constructed as shown in Figure 2-6. For any one body fat, the endurance of the women was always greater than that of the men. However, for both groups of subjects there was a dramatic reduction in endurance as the body fat was increased. One problem with these earlier studies was in the estimation of body fat. Ideal height and weight tables are inherently incorrect for the individual, although they do seem to be acceptable for large populations. Therefore, an additional series of experiments was conducted to examine further the relationship between body fat and isometric endurance. In these studies, body fat was measured by underwater weight as described by Keys and Brozek (1953). Here a smaller group of subjects was used, and isometric contractions were again performed with the handgrip muscles at a tension of 40 percent MVC. As described for the large population, there was an inverse relationship between body fat and isometric endurance (Petrofsky and Lind 1975).

The mechanism of this response appeared to be related once again to the temperature of the exercising muscles. When Petrofsky and Lind (1975) measured the muscle temperature of the brachioradialis muscle in eight subjects, there was a direct relationship between the temperature of the brachioradialis muscle at rest and the body fat of the subjects (*See* Figure 2-7). In further studies (Petrofsky and Lind 1975), they found that weight loss or weight gain would reduce or increase the resting muscle temperature, respectively, and reversibly alter isometric endurance. It appeared, then, that the changes in muscle temperature were of a sufficient magnitude in the overweight to account for the reduced isometric endurance. Therefore, in a final series of experiments, several subjects gained and lost weight, and their isometric endurance was measured once again. Here, however, isometric endurance was measured after the subjects had immersed their arms in a water bath for thirty minutes. With muscle temperature stabilized before and after weight loss, there was no difference in the isometric endurance with weight loss or weight gain.

These experiments were repeated in a later series of experiments during which isometric contractions of the handgrip muscles were sustained at tensions of 25, 40, 55, and 70 percent MVC, and similar results were found for all tensions examined (Petrofsky and Phillips 1981). However, the largest difference in isometric endurance between thin and overweight subjects was

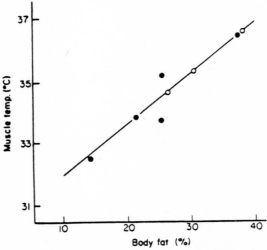

Figure 2-7.   Relation of deep muscle temperature at 40 percent of the distance between the skin and the center of the forearm to the percentage of body fat in three male (○) and five female (●) subjects. From Petrofsky and Lind, The Relationship of Body Fat Content to Deep Muscle Temperature, *Clin Sci Mol Med*, *48*:405–412, 1975. Courtesy of Biochemical Society.

found for contractions at the lowest isometric tensions. For example, when comparing the effect of muscle temperature on isometric endurance for contractions at 25 and 70 percent MVC, it was found that as the muscle temperature was changed from 28°–38° C the endurance in a group of eight subjects tripled, whereas isometric endurance was only increased about 1.5-fold over the same range of muscle temperatures for contractions exerted at 70 percent MVC (Petrofsky and Phillips 1981).

Strength and Endurance

Although the relationship between strength and endurance has been well established in the literature, it has been controversial as to the exact relationship between strength and endurance. Elbel (1949), Tuttle and Horvath (1957), Cotton (1970),

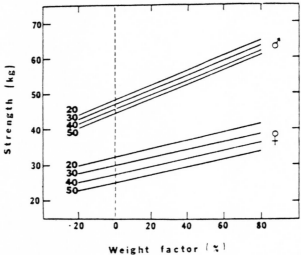

Figure 2-8.   Multifactor analysis of the relationship of strength to age and body weight factor in men (upper curves) and women (lower curves). Here, strength (ordinate) *i* related to the body weight (abscissa) with four individual lines calculated for individuals 20, 30, 40, and 50 years of age. The multiple regression equations are: $y (\pm 6.9) = 51.59 - 0.206$ wt for males and $y (\pm 5.4) = 37.9 - 0.247$ age $+ 0.107$ wt for females. From Petrofsky and Lind, Isometric Strength, Endurance and the Blood Pressure and Heart Rate, *Europ J Physiol, 360*:49–61, 1975. Courtesy of Springer Verlag New York, Inc.

Josenhans (1962), and Start and Graham (1964) all showed a negative correlation between strength and relative endurance. In contrast, Shaver (1972), Rohmert (1968), and Caldwell (1964) all found no significant correlation between static strength and relative endurance. In the work cited previously (Petrofsky and Lind 1975), we also found a negative correlation between grip strength and relative endurance. However, there was a positive correlation between grip strength and body fat (*See* Figure 2-8). Since isometric endurance is lower in the overweight, due to an increase in muscle temperature, the negative correlation between grip strength and endurance was shown to be related to body fat and not grip strength per se. When individuals of various strengths were matched for body fat, there was no significant

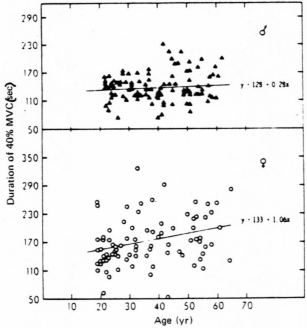

Figure 2-9. Duration of a 40 percent MVC isometric contraction in seconds for each of the 100 males (▲) and 83 females (○) of different ages. Regression lines are illustrated for each sex. From Petrofsky, Burse, and Lind, Comparison of Physiological Responses of Women and Men to Isometric Exercise, *J Appl Physiol 38*:863–868, 1975. Courtesy of The American Physiological Society.

correlation between strength and endurance. Rohmert and Caldwell used matched subjects in their studies. In contrast, Elbel (1949), Tuttle and Horvath (1957), and Josenhans (1962) examined subjects with a wide variety of body compositions; this then may account for differences in these results.

Sex Differences

One surprising finding in some of the studies described in this chapter (Petrofsky, Burse, and Lind 1975), and which was confirmed later (Heyward and McCreory 1977), was that the female subjects had longer isometric endurance at *any* body fat than the male subjects. When this was examined further, it was found that, even in matched population of male and female subjects

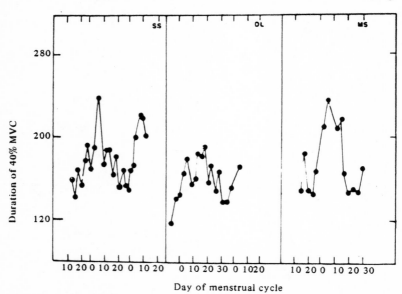

Figure 2-10. The endurance of the first of five successive fatiguing contractions at 40 percent MVC for each of three "normal" subjects over two months is illustrated here (N. B. the days of the menstrual cycle shown on the abscissa start on different days of the cycle for each subject just as they occurred experimentally.) From Petrofsky et al., Isometric Strength and Endurance During the Menstrual Cycle in Healthy Young Women, *Eur J Appl Physiol, 35*:1–10, 1976. Courtesy of Springer-Verlag New York, Inc.

(matched in terms of age and body fat), the women usually had about one-third longer endurance than their male counterparts for contractions at a tension of 40 percent MVC with the hand-grip muscles (Petrofsky and Lind 1975). Further examination of this phenomena showed that the greatest difference in endurance between men and women occurred in the youngest age groups (i.e. 15–35 years old) (*See* Figure 2-9).

It was also found that the variability in endurance to sustain contractions at 40 percent MVC in the female subjects was much greater than those of their male counterparts. The logical conclusion of these studies was that some of the difference in endurance was related to sex hormones. Since sex hormones vary in concentration throughout the menstrual cycle in the female subjects, this might also explain the greater variability in endur-

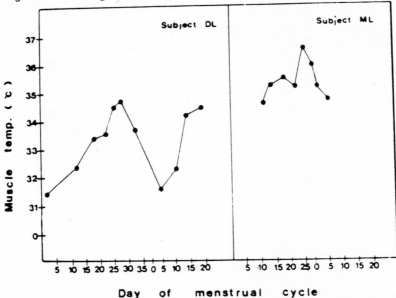

Figure 2-11.   The temperature of the bracheoradialus muscle measured at 40 percent of the distance between the skin and center of the forearm for two control subjects during one menstrual cycle are illustrated here. From Petrofsky et al., Isometric Strength and Endurance During the Menstrual Cycle in Healthy Young Women, *Eur J Appl Physiol*, 35:1–10, 1976. Courtesy of Springer-Verlag New York, Inc.

ance recorded in these subjects. Therefore, a series of experiments was conducted to examine further the isometric endurance in female subjects. Six female subjects participated in these experiments to look at the isometric endurance of the handgrip muscles at a tension of 40 percent throughout the menstrual cycle. Three of the subjects were on the birth control pill and three had normal menstrual cycles (controls). The results of these experiments showed that in the women not taking the birth control pill there was a sinusoidal variation in endurance throughout the menstrual cycle (*See* Figure 2-10) (Petrofsky et al. 1976). The longest isometric endurance occurred at about the seventh day after the onset of bleeding, while the lowest isometric endurance occurred at about the twenty-second day after the onset of bleeding. The total variation in endurance over this period was about thirty percent. The women taking the birth control pill always had less endurance than the controls and had little variation in their endurance throughout the menstrual cycle. It was found later that menopausal women also had less endurance than women having a normal menstrual cycle and had no variation in isometric endurance over the period of the month. It therefore appeared that sex hormones were in some way related to isometric endurance. Part of this variation in endurance could be attributed to changes in deep muscle temperature, since it was also shown that there were fluctuations in the forearm resting muscle temperatures of the control subjects of as much as 2° C throughout the menstrual cycle; this variation did not occur in women taking the birth control pill (*See* Figure 2-11). However, even when the muscle temperature of the controls was stabilized throughout the menstrual cycle, there was still some variation in isometric endurance that could not be accounted for. The mechanism of this response is still obscure, since the endurance of the controls did not cycle and phase with any known hormone.

Age

Another factor that has a large influence on isometric endurance for a single sustained submaximal isometric contraction is age. When the isometric endurance was measured in men and women whose ages ranged from 18–72 years for a contraction at

40 percent MVC of the handgrip muscles, it was found that, although aging was associated with a reduction in strength, there was a marked increase in isometric endurance in both male and female subjects (*See* Figure 2-9). In both the male and female subjects that were examined, an increase in age from the second to the fifth decade of life resulted in a corresponding increase in isometric endurance by 12 percent, and 28 percent in male and female subjects, respectively; these studies were confirmed later by Larsson and Karlsson (1978). It was felt that the mechanism of this response was related to the fiber composition of the muscles.

At birth, all muscles have similar fiber compositions. Muscles are composed of an embryonic type of muscle, which resembles the slow-twitch muscle of the adult (Gutman and Hanzlekova 1972). However, within a few days after birth, muscles differentiate into the fast-twitch and slow-twitch motor units of the adult (Buller et al. 1969; Close 1964; Denny-Brown 1929; Drahota and Gutman 1963; Hajek et al. 1963). Although this differentiation takes place at an early age, no further changes occur until the middle of the second decade of life. At this point, motor units are lost due to destruction in the central nervous system, and the remaining muscle fibers begin to slowly dedifferentiate back into slow-twitch motor units (Gutman and Hanzlekova 1972; Larsson and Karlsson 1978; Larsson et al. 1979). This process can be retarded to some extent by physical training, but even in well-trained athletes the process still occurs. Classically, slow-twitch motor units are associated with low strength and high endurance. In contrast, fast-twitch motor units are associated with high strength but low isometric endurance. It is not surprising then that aging would be associated with a reduction in isometric strength and an increase in isometric endurance.

Fast and Slow Muscle

Although the relationship between strength and endurance in fast- and slow-twitch motor units has been examined during tetanic contractions in skeletal muscle in many type of animals (Close 1972, Burke et al. 1965), the exact relationship between strength and endurance in fast- and slow-twitch motor units has never been established. It would be very difficult in man to separate fast- and slow-twitch motor units and study the strength-endurance relationship since muscles in man are predominately mixed in terms of their fiber composition.

To a limited extent, the fast-and slow-twitch motor units can be blocked differentially by decamethonium (which blocks fast-twitch motor units) and curare (which blocks slow-twitch motor units) (Molbech and Johansen 1969). If these drugs are infused into man, isometric endurance is much shorter in fast-twitch than slow-twitch motor units (Molbech and Johansen 1969). However, these experiments were limited due to the fact that total block could not be achieved with drugs.

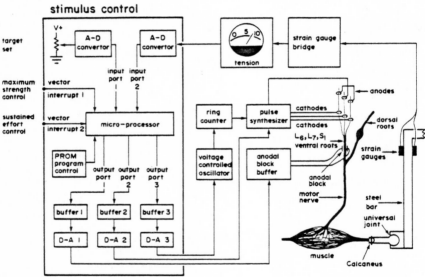

Figure 2-12.   Schematic representation of the computer-controlled stimulation system. Muscles are stimulated through bundles of the appropriate ventral roots of the spinal cord by a pulse-synthesizer network. Tension, generated by the muscle, is transduced by a pair of strain gauges mounted on a steel tension bar to an electrical output, which provide the computer with feedback information of muscle tension. From Petrofsky, Control of the Recruitment and Firing Frequencies of Motor Units in Electrically Stimulated Muscles in the Cat, *Med Biol Eng, 16*:302–308, 1978. Courtesy of Medical and Biological Engineering and Computing.

One recurrent problem that often occurs in animal experimentation is that muscles are stimulated by a very artificial means. Typically, muscles are stimulated by a single pair of electrodes applied to either the motor nerve or the muscle at stimulation voltages and frequencies far in excess of the normal physiological range (Petrofsky 1978). However, many muscles in animals are either pure fast- or pure slow-twitch (Ariano et al. 1973). Therefore, it would be a substantial advantage to examine the strength endurance relationship in these muscles. We therefore attempted to devise a stimulation technique that would allow us to stimulate the muscle in a more physiological manner and, at the same time, to control tension development very precisely during sustained submaximal isometric contractions. Rack and Westbury (1969) found that the normal asynchronous mode of motor unit recruitment found during voluntary activity could be mimicked by sequential stimulation of as little as three groups of motor units; this was confirmed in our own work (Lind and Petrofsky 1979). The principle advantage of sequential motor unit stimulation is that it allows motor units to fully tetanize at stimulation frequencies as low as 40 Hz. This frequency is within the normal physiological range. In contrast, to tetanize muscle fully during stimulation with a single pair of electrodes requires stimulation frequencies between 100 Hz and 300 Hz — a stimulation frequency far outside the normal physiological range. Using this form of stimulation, then, we developed a microprocessor-controlled stimulator as shown in Figure 2-12.

The stimulator accomplishes several things. First of all, the stimulator enabled us to sequentially stimulate the motor units in the muscle. The motor units in the muscle used in these studies (soleus, medial gastrocnemius, and the plantaris muscles of the cat) were stimulated through the ventral roots of the spinal cord (L6, L7, S1). These three sets of ventral roots contain the entire alpha efferent innervation to these muscles. The three groups of ventral roots were first pooled together surgically and then subdivided into three bundles, which were stimulated sequentially. These muscles were chosen since the soleus muscle in the cat is a pure slow-twitch muscle, while the medial gastrocnemius and plantaris are mixed but predominately fast-twitch muscles

(Ariano et al. 1973). To set the recruitment order in the same manner as occurs during voluntary activity (Bigland and Lippold 1954; Milner-Brown and Stein 1975) (*see* Chapter 3 *isometric contractions*), initially, all motor units were recruited by applying a sufficient stimulating voltage to develop action potentials in all

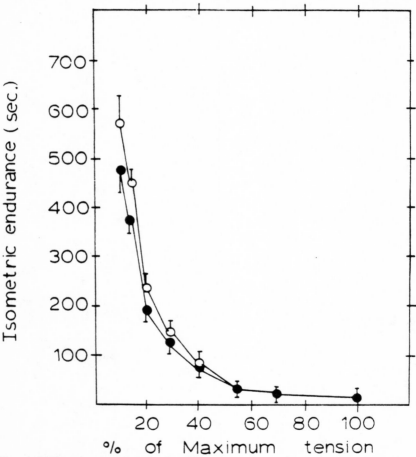

Figure 2-13.   Average isometric endurance in the medial gastrocnemius muscle of four cats (●) compared to four human subjects (○). From Petrofsky and Phillips, Microprocessor Stimulation of Paralyzed Muscle, © 1979 *IEEE*, 198–210. Reprinted with permission from proceedings of the IEEE 1979 National Aerospace and Electronics Conference, NAECON 1979, Volume 1, May 15-17, 1979, Dayton, Ohio.

the alpha motor neurons by the three sequential electrodes. These action potentials were blocked by an anodal block electrode. To vary recruitment in the muscle, the anodal block voltage was removed gradually. As the anodal block voltage was removed, motor units that were less susceptible to an anodal block were recruited first. Since slow-twitch motor units are less susceptible to anodal blockade, the order of motor unit recruitment was from the slowest to fastest motor units respectively (Petrofsky 1978, 1979; Petrofsky and Lind 1979). This is the normal order of motor unit recruitment that has been observed in man and animal experiments (Bigland and Lippold 1954; Milner-Brown and Stein 1975). The pattern of stimulation used during sustained isometric contractions is also based on those reported to occur in man. At the onset of a fatiguing isometric contraction, the initial tension developed by the muscle was achieved by a combination of first recruitment and then changes in the firing frequency of the motor units (rate coding). Initially, all motor units were recruited at a frequency of 10 Hz. Motor unit recruitment was used to vary tension from 0-50 percent of the initial strength of the muscles (tetanic tension). For tensions greater than 50 percent of the initial strength, all motor units were initially recruited, and the discharge frequency of the motor units was increased until the target tension was reached. As the contractions were sustained, due to motor unit fatigue, the tension began to fall. This fall in tension was sensed by the strain gauge bridge, which monitored tension developed by the muscle, and the computer in turn compensated for the fall in tension by increasing either recruitment or the discharge frequency of the motor units. When an increase in frequency of discharge was no longer effective in maintaining the target, the contraction was terminated, and the entire length of time the contraction was sustained was called the endurance time. In this manner, then, it was possible to use an animal model to simulate normal sustained voluntary isometric contractions. The medial gastrocnemius muscle in the cat has an isometric endurance similar to that which occurs in the forearm muscles of man (*See* Figure 2-13). Like the muscles in man, the medial gastrocnemius muscle — a mixed muscle — can sustain tensions up to about 10 percent of its initial strength without fatiguing. Above these tensions the muscle begins to fatigue rapidly.

The isometric endurance of the soleus muscle (a pure slow-twitch muscle) and the plantaris muscle (a fast-twitch muscle with some slow-twitch motor units) was in sharp contrast to those observed for the medial gastrocnemius. For the soleus, although the general shape of the strength endurance curve was the same as those reported for the medial gastrocnemius muscle and for man, it was found that the soleus muscle could sustain contraction tensions of up to about 30 percent of its isometric strength with no sign of muscle fatigue (*See* Figure 2-14). For contractions at tensions above this, although the muscle fatigued, there was still a substantially longer isometric endurance than that which was found for the medial gastrocnemius muscle at all tensions examined.

The effect of muscle temperature on the contractile characteristics of fast- and slow-twitch muscle is also different. Close

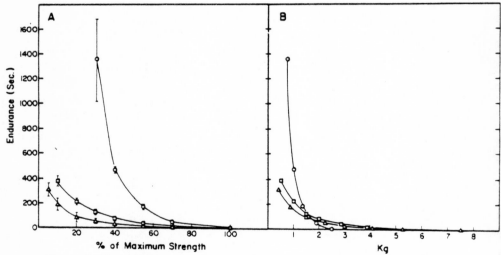

Figure 2-14.   Average isometric endurance recorded for plantaris (△), gastrocnemius (□), and soleus (○) in the cat in relation to both relative (A) and absolute (B) tension exerted by muscles. Each point shows mean endurance ± SD of four muscles studied. From Petrofsky and Lind, Isometric Endurance in Fast and Slow Muscles, *Am J Physiol, 236*:185–191, 1979. Courtesy of The American Physiological Society.

and Hoh (1968) found that the tetanic tension developed by slow-twitch muscle does not vary appreciably over the temperature range of 38° to 28° C. Below 28° C muscle temperature and tetanic tension were directly related to each other. In contrast, in a fast-twitch muscle, they found that tetanic tension was reduced at all temperatures below 38° C. In a similar manner, the effect of muscle temperature on isometric endurance also varies with the fiber composition of the muscles. Whereas the isometric endurance in a mixed muscle in man or in the cat shows a twofold increase in endurance when cooled from 38° to 28° C, the endurance of fast-twitch muscles is constant over this same range of muscle temperatures, while slow-twitch muscle triples its endurance under similar circumstances. Both types of muscle show a reduction in endurance at temperatures below 28° C (Petrofsky and Lind 1981).

Blood Flow

Gaskell (1877) first described the hyperemia following exercise. The blood flow through muscle during isometric exercise can influence the endurance for isometric contractions. Lind et al. (1964) demonstrated that due to high intramuscular pressure, the blood flow was occluded in contracting handgrip muscles at tensions greater than 70 percent MVC. It is not surprising then that isometric endurance of the handgrip muscles is not different if the circulation to the muscle is occluded for contractions greater than 70 percent MVC (Simonson 1972; Lind et al. 1978). For contractions less than 70 percent MVC, occlusion reduces isometric endurance. This same relationship holds for many other muscles (Start and Graham 1964; Royce 1957; Kearny et al. 1976; McGlynn and McCreary 1969; Heyward 1977; Serfess et al. 1979; Edwards et al. 1977). Muscles with a high composition of slow-twitch motor units appear to be more susceptible to occlusion than muscles with a high, fast-twitch fiber population (Petrofsky and Lind 1979; Petrofsky et al. 1981) due to the heavy dependance of slow-twitch motor units on blood flow (Close 1972; Folkow and Halicka 1968). Further, in some muscles, blood flow is occluded at lower tensions due presumably to a nipping of the arteries to the muscle by muscle contractions (Barcroft and Millen 1939). For the calf muscles, occlusion of the circulation occurs for contractions greater than 30 percent MVC.

Recovery of Endurance

The endurance for isometric exercise takes about twenty-four hours to fully recover following a fatiguing isometric contraction (Kroll 1968; Edwards et al. 1977; Funderburk et al. 1974; Petrofsky and Phillips 1981; Stafford and Petrofsky 1981). However, although recovery is slow following isometric exercise; most of the recovery is over within twenty minutes after the exercise. For example, following a contraction at 40 percent MVC, if a second contraction is performed at the same tension twenty minutes later, the endurance of the second contraction

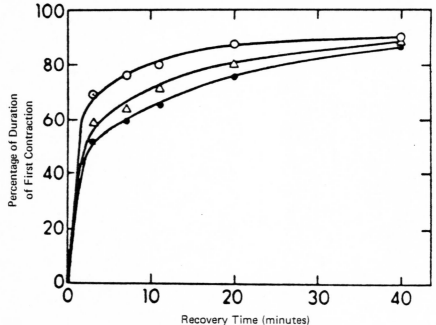

Figure 2-15. Recovery of the ability of muscles to sustain static effort at 20 (•), 40 (△) and 60 (○) MVC after fatiguing contractions, expressed as percentage of duration of the first contraction at each tension. From Funderburk et al., The Development of and Recovery from Muscular Fatigue Induced by Static Effort at Different Tensions, *J Appl Physiol, 37*:392–401, 1974. Courtesy of The American Physiological Society.

will be about 80 percent that of the first. Funderburk et al. (1974) found that the fastest rate of recovery following fatiguing isometric contractions occurred for contractions at high isometric tensions (*See* Figure 2-15). This has been confirmed in a number of later studies.

If the isometric contractions are sustained for periods of time less than that necessary to bring the muscle to fatigue, then the recovery is even somewhat faster. The interrelationship between the length of sustained contractions and the length of the rest

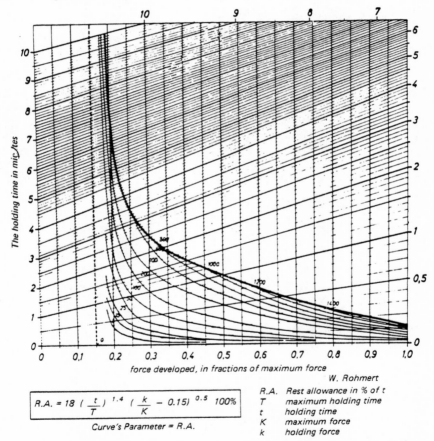

W. Rohmert

$$R.A. = 18 \left(\frac{t}{T} \right)^{1.4} \left(\frac{k}{K} - 0.15 \right)^{0.5} 100\%$$

Curve's Parameter = R.A.

R.A.	Rest allowance in % of t
T	maximum holding time
t	holding time
K	maximum force
k	holding force

Figure 2-16.   Rest allowances for static work. From W. Rohmert, Ermittlung von Erholungspausen für Statische Arbeit des Menschen. *Int Z Agnew Physiol, 8*:123–127; 1960. Courtesy of Springer-Verlag New York, Inc.

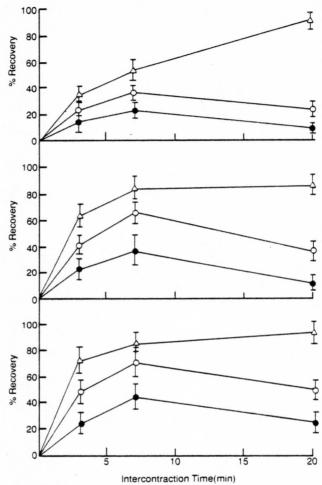

Figure 2-17. The percent recovery (the endurance of the second contraction normalized to the endurance of first contraction) recorded from eight subjects for contractions at tensions of 25 percent (upper panel), 40 percent (middle panel), and 70 percent MVC (lower panel) with an intercontraction time interval of 3, 7, or 10 mins. During non-fatiguing contraction of 5 (○) or 10 percent (△). Each point in this figure shows the mean response of the group ± SD. From Stafford and Petrofsky, the Relationship Between Fatiguing and Non-fatiguing Isometric Contractions, *J Appl Physiol, 51*:399–404, 1981. Courtesy of Journal of Applied Physiology.

pauses in between contractions was described by Rohmert and is shown in Figure 2-16.

Muscle temperature has some effect of recovery following isometric exercise. In recent work, we found that when comparing the recovery from fatiguing isometric contractions at muscle temperatures of 28°–38° C, although the recovery was the same for contractions longer than seven-minute intervals, the recovery of endurance was somewhat faster at the warmer muscle temperature for contractions separated by intervals of less than seven minutes (Petrofsky and Phillips 1981).

Although contractions at tensions less than 15 percent MVC are considered to be non-fatiguing, contractions of these light isometric tensions in the recovery interval following fatiguing isometric contractions can dramatically reduce recovery. If a contraction at 5 or 10 percent MVC is sustained for as long as twenty minutes prior to a fatiguing isometric contraction, there is no difference in the endurance of the fatiguing isometric contraction when comparing these endurance times for those of the previously uncontracted muscle. However, when contractions are sustained at these non-fatiguing tensions following a fatiguing isometric contraction, recovery is reduced in proportion to both the length the non-fatiguing contraction is held and in proportion to the tension exerted by the muscle. For example, in Figure 2-17, it can be seen that for eight male subjects, although recovery was 80 percent complete when contractions were sustained with intervals of twenty minutes when no exercise was done in between the contractions, if a fatiguing isometric contraction was sustained during the intercontraction interval at 5 or 10 percent MVC, the recovery was only 25 and 30 percent complete for the second isometric contraction. Generally, fatiguing contractions at the lowest isometric tensions were associated with the greatest reduction in recovery when submaximal non-fatiguing isometric tensions were sustained during the recovery interval. Since it is very common to mix fatiguing and non-fatiguing isometric contractions in an industrial setting, these findings are particularly relevant to work physiology.

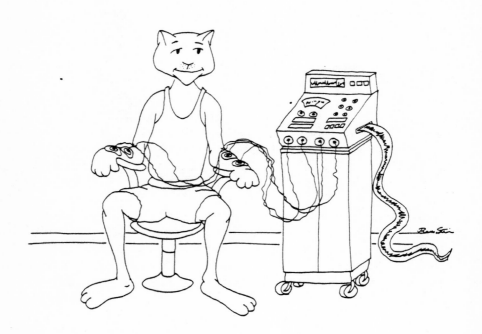

CHAPTER 3

MOTOR UNIT RECRUITMENT PATTERNS AND THE ELECTROMYOGRAM DURING STATIC EFFORT

MOTOR UNIT RECRUITMENT DURING STATIC EFFORT

During isometric contractions the tension developed by muscle can be graded by one of two means. Tension can be adjusted by the central nervous system by either changing the number of motor units that are recruited or by altering the frequency of discharge of previously recruited motor units. From studies of brief isometric contractions, it has been found in man (Bigland and Lippold 1954; Edwards and Lippold 1956; Milner-Brown and Stein 1975; Monster 1979; Kosarov et al. 1979; Clamann 1970) and in the cat (Olson et al. 1968) that for tensions up to about 50 percent of a muscle's maximum strength, the tension is adjusted by varying motor unit recruitment. Over this range of tensions, once a motor unit is recruited, its frequency of discharge remains fairly constant while other motor units are recruited. For example, as shown in Figure 3-1, it can be seen that different motor units are recruited at various tensions. The frequency of motor unit discharge at the time of recruitment usually varies between 5 Hz and 15 Hz and remains somewhat constant until the tension exceeds 50 percent of the muscles maximum strength (Milner-Brown and Stein 1975). Once the tension developed by the muscle exceeds about half of its maximum strength, all motor units have been recruited. As the tension developed by the muscle is increased from 50 to 100 percent of the muscle's strength, motor unit discharge frequencies are used to vary tension. The highest discharge frequencies found usually averaged between 40 Hz and 60 Hz during a maximal effort.

37

Motor units are not recruited in a random fashion. In both human and animal experiments, it has been shown that motor units are generally recruited by size from the smallest to largest, respectively (Olson et al. 1968). Since the smallest motor nerves are those associated with slow-twitch motor units within the muscle, it has been concluded that slow-twitch motor units are recruited first. Slow-twitch motor units are associated with less strength but greater endurance than are fast-twitch motor units (Close 1972). This makes good sense, since light isometric contractions are commonly associated with activity such as holding a pencil or other light objects. These contractions can be sustained for long periods of time without any sign of muscle fatigue. Although this order of recruitment is typically seen in both animal (Olson et al. 1968) and human experiments (Milner-Brown and Stein 1975; Grimby and Hannerz 1976; Hannerz and Grimby 1979), previous physical activity can alter the normal pattern of motor unit recruitment. For example, Grimby and Hannerz (1976) and Hannerz and Grimby (1979) have shown that the

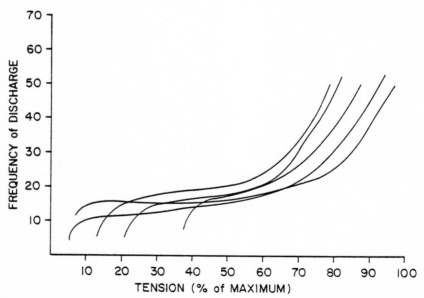

Figure 3-1.   Discharge frequency and onset of recruitment in different motor units in the adductor polysis muscle in man during voluntary contractions at tensions up to 100 percent MVC.

proprioceptive activity can alter the afferent discharge pattern to skeletal muscle thereby altering the pattern of motor unit recruitment. Motor unit recruitment also is different during fast phasic isometric contractions as compared to sustained effort.

Although the pattern of motor unit recruitment has been well described during brief isometric contractions, much less is known during sustained isometric contractions. What little is known suggests that during sustained isometric contractions the pattern of motor unit recruitment and frequency of discharge parallels that which occurs during brief isometric contractions (Petrofsky 1981). At the onset of the sustained or fatiguing isometric contractions, motor units are initially recruited as described here for brief isometric contractions. However, as the contraction is sustained, due to fatigue of the recruited motor units, the tension developed by the muscle will diminish. To sustain the target tension held during the contraction, the central nervous system either increases recruitment of motor units (if all motor units have not been recruited) or increases the frequency of discharge of motor units (once all motor units have been recruited). This procedure is continued by the central nervous system until the contraction is terminated. Clearly, however, isometric contractions can be subdivided into two types: submaximal isometric contractions and sustained maximal effort. The pattern of motor unit recruitment and frequency of discharge as described here pertains to sustained submaximal isometric contractions. During a sustained maximal effort (contraction where a subject continually exerts maximal effort while, due to fatigue, the tension continues to fall) a different pattern of motor unit recruitment is found. At the onset of a contraction, all motor units are initially recruited and the frequency of discharge approaches 60 Hz - 70 Hz. Obviously, no further recruitment can take place. What appears to occur is that as the tension is sustained, motor units fatigue. Associated with this fatigue is a rapid fall in the tension developed by the muscle. In parallel with this fall in tension is a fall in the discharge frequency of motor units (Bigland-Richie and Lippold 1980). This phenomena is described in more detail later in this chapter.

THE ELECTROMYOGRAM

The surface electromyogram is a complex interference pattern arising from active muscle. If a pair of electrodes are placed on the skin overlying a muscle and several muscle fibers discharge randomly, the action potential can be recorded from the skin (*See* Figure 3-2). The surface recording will appear as that shown in panel A of this figure. In contrast, if three muscle fibers discharge in phase with one another, as shown in panel B of this figure, the action potentials will summate in the surface recording. Muscle fibers rarely fire either independently or synchronously. An alpha motor neuron innervates as many as 6,000 muscle fibers; this structure comprising a single motor unit. Because the point of innervation of muscle fibers within a motor unit is slightly different, action potentials arising on the various muscle fibers within the motor unit arrive under the recording electrodes slightly out of phase with one another. The result of this can be demonstrated in panel C of this figure and represents a motor unit action potential (MUAP). The electrical wave recorded on the surface during voluntary discharge of hundreds of motor units reflects the algebraic summation of the individual MUAP's of each of the motor units. The wave is longer in duration than any of the individual muscle fiber action potentials. Under most everyday activities, motor units fire out of phase with one another, although some synchronization has been found in some experiments between the discharge of various

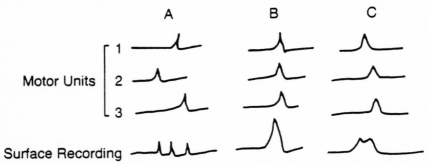

Figure 3-2.   Surface recording of the EMG during random (A) and synchronized (B) firing of three motor units. Panel C illustrates a motor unit action potential (MUAP).

motor units (Milner-Brown and Stein 1975). The result is obvious: Since motor units fire out of phase with one another, the algebraic summation of the individual motor unit potentials as shown in Figure 3-3 is a complex wave reflecting the algebraic summation of all the random discharges of the motor units in a muscle. This complex wave, when recorded from the surface of the skin, is called the *surface electromyogram* or *surface EMG*.

The Amplitude of the Surface EMG

I. Brief Contractions

The amplitude of the electromyogram can be measured by a number of different means. Since the wave is symmetrical around zero, the amplitude can be assessed by measuring either the average peak amplitude of the complex waves, the average half- or full-wave amplitude of the EMG (rectified EMG), the integrated amplitude of the EMG (area under the wave), or by

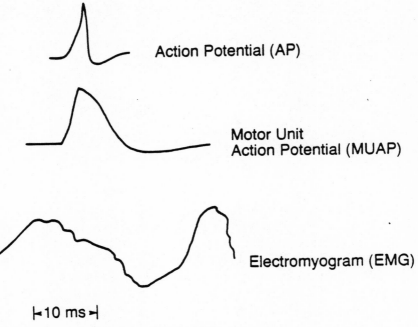

Figure 3-3.   Genesis of the surface EMG.

measuring the RMS amplitude of the EMG (root-mean-square). When subjects are asked to exert brief isometric contractions at tensions between 5 and 100 percent of their maximum voluntary strength, it has been found by many (Lippold 1952; Bigland and Lippold 1954; Edwards and Lippold 1956; Milner-Brown and Stein 1975; Kurodn et al. 1970; Petrofsky et al. 1976; Lind and Petrofsky 1979; Petrofsky 1980) investigators that the relationship between the amplitude of the EMG (measured by any of the means as previously described) and tension is linear, as shown in Figure 3-4. However, although most investigators have reported this relationship to be linear in some experiments, investigators have found non-linearities in this relationship to exist at either high or low isometric tensions (Zuniga and Simmons 1969). This non-linearity may be due to a number of different sources. One of the most common sources is in the design of the dynamometer used to measure the tension. It is important that the dynamometer only exercise the muscles being tested. If other muscle groups begin to contract at high or low tensions, this will be detected by the surface EMG electrodes and result in non-linearities in the EMG tension relationship. The pattern of recruitment used to activate the muscle may also cause non-linearities. As described previously, prior activity in the muscle or proprioceptive activity from muscle afferents can alter the normal patterns of motor unit recruitment. This in turn might alter the EMG tension relationship. Finally, it has been shown that electrode placement is very important in determining the EMG tension relationship (Lynn 1978). When electrodes are placed more than 4 cm apart over an active muscle, the EMG tension relationship typically becomes non-linear, especially at the higher isometric tensions. In some experiments, where non-linearity has been reported, electrodes have been spaced at very wide distances. However, it must be stressed that most studies do report a linear relationship between EMG amplitude and tension for brief isometric contractions.

This phenomenon has always been somewhat surprising since it has been shown by Bigland and Lippold (1954) that recruitment is complete for contractions at tensions above 50 percent of the maximum voluntary strength. Tension is adjusted for con-

tractions above 50 percent of the maximum voluntary strength
by altering the firing frequency of the previously recruited
motor units. However, Milner-Brown and Stein (1975) in an ex-

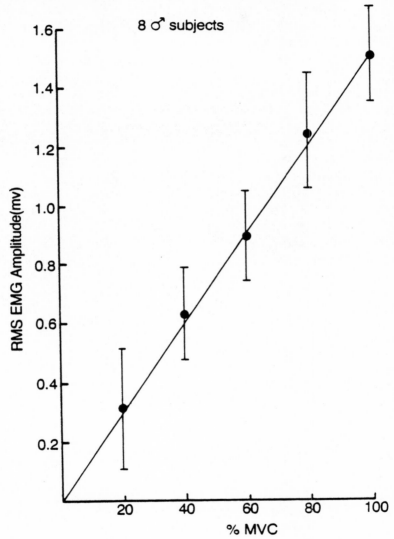

Figure 3-4. The relationship between the amplitude of the EMG and tension
during brief (3 seconds) isometric contractions of the handgrip
muscles in four subjects.

tensive study of the EMG tension relationship found that recruitment and adjustments of motor unit firing frequency,
which they termed "rate coding," contributed equally to the
amplitude of the surface-recorded EMG. Therefore, equal increments in rate coding or recruitment could cause the same increase in the amplitude of the surface EMG. This explains the
linear relationship between tension and amplitude of the surface
EMG.

One problem encountered in these studies, however, was the
fact that although the relationship between EMG amplitude and
tension was linear for any one individual, there is a large degree
of variability in the EMG amplitude for contractions sustained at
one given tension, not only between individuals, but within the
same individual from day to day (*See* Figure 3-4). For this reason,
it has become a common practice in EMG studies to normalize
the amplitude of the EMG (as will be done in the remainder of
this chapter) in terms of the EMG amplitude during an MVC
(maximal voluntary contraction). When this occurs, the variability is reduced dramatically, as shown in Figure 3-5. Some of this

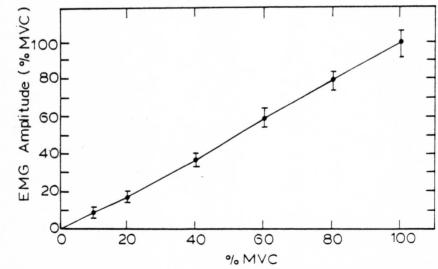

Figure 3-5.   The relationship between the normalized amplitude of the EMG
and tension during brief (3 seconds) isometric contractions of the
handgrip muscles of the four subjects, as shown in Figure 3-4.

variability in the absolute level of the EMG amplitude from day to day must certainly lie in variations in the recording electrodes and electrode placement. But even when electrodes are matched in terms of impedance characteristics and are placed in the same spot from day to day, although the variability is reduced dramatically, some variability still occurs. One factor that might cause some of this variability is muscle temperature.

Unlike the temperature of the core of the body, the temperature of the shell tissues is not regulated closely. The shell tissues of the body are used as a heat exchange device to help regulate the temperature of the core tissues. When core temperature rises, blood flow is increased to the shell tissues to allow for greater heat exchange with the environment. In contrast, when core temperature is low, blood flow is restricted to the shell tissues, allowing for the conservation of heat. For this reason, the temperature of the shell tissues may vary by as much as 10° C or more from that of the core. Most skeletal muscles in the body are located in the shell. For this reason, the temperature of most skeletal muscles is quite variable from day to day. The brachioradialus muscle of the forearm, for example, generally has a resting muscle temperature of 32° C in a subject exposed to a comfortable environment with his arms bared to the shoulder (Barcroft and Edhohm 1943; Clarke, Hellon, and Lind 1958; Petrofsky and Lind 1975). In contrast, in a cool or warm environment, the muscle temperature may be as low as 22° C or as high as 38° C. Muscle temperature in turn can affect the amplitude of the EMG. When muscle temperature is varied between 28° and 38° C, for example, by immersing the forearm of subjects in a water bath for thirty minutes prior to the contractions, the amplitude of the EMG during an MVC is found to be inversely related to muscle temperature (*See* Figure 3-6) (Petrofsky 1980; Petrofsky and Lind 1980). In addition, if the EMG tension relationship is in itself measured at various muscle temperatures (*See* Figure 3-7), the EMG tension relationship becomes non-linear at cooler muscle temperatures. Therefore, normal physiological variations in the temperature of contracting skeletal muscles may account for some of the non-linearities in the EMG tension relationship as well as variations in the absolute magnitude of the EMG seen in different experiments. The mechanism of these variations appears to be related to changes in the electrical characteristics of the sarcolemma and to variations in recruitment of motor units associated with altering muscle temperature. Measurement of the impedance of the skin and between the skin and muscle do show an inverse relationship between impedance and skin and muscle temperature (*See* Figure 3-8). However, if a signal is injected into a muscle, when the skin and muscle temperature is varied over a 10° C range, and

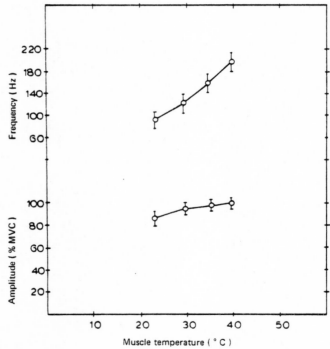

Figure 3-6.   The relationship between the RMS amplitude and center frequency of the EMG power spectra and muscle temperature during a brief isometric contraction at 100 percent MVC in each of four subjects. Each point illustrates the mean of two experiments ± the SD on each of the subjects. From Petrofsky, Frequency and Amplitude Analysis of the EMG During Exercise on the Bicycle Ergometer, *Eur J Appl Physiol, 41*:1–15, 1979. Courtesy of Springer-Verlag New York, Inc.

muscle blood flow is varied over a ten-fold range due to hyperemia induced by anoxia, the signal transmitted from the muscle to the skin is not attenuated (*See* Figure 3-10).

Another source of variation in the amplitude of the EMG and the EMG tension relationship could also be the length of the muscles prior to isometric contraction. For example, extending the arm and thereby changing the angle between the forearm and upper arm causes a large change in the length of the biceps and triceps muscles. This stretches the sarcolemma (muscle cell membrane) and causes the electrical characteristics of the membrane to change dramatically (Kaiser and Peterson 1963). Further, muscle strength varies widely over the same range of muscle lengths (Petrofsky and Phillips 1980). For example, by passively moving the forearm to allow the angle of the elbow to vary between 30° and 170°, and measuring the maximum isometric strength, it is found that the optimal elbow angle for performing an isometric contraction is at an angle of about 120°. In contrast, the absolute EMG amplitude at all elbow angles stays

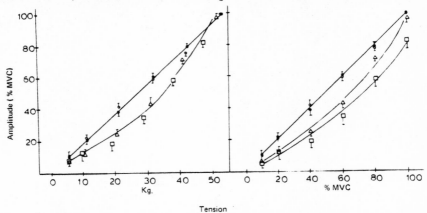

Tension

Figure 3-7.   The RMS amplitude of the power spectra of the surface EMG during brief isometric contractions at each of four bath temperatures, 10° (□), 20° (△), 30° (○), and 40° (●) C compared to both the relative and absolute tension developed by the muscles. Each point illustrates the mean of two experiments on each of ten subjects ± SD. From Petrofsky and Lind, the Influence of Temperature on the Amplitude and Frequency Components, *Eur J Appl Physiol*, *44*:189–200, 1980. Courtesy of Springer-Verlag New York Inc.

fairly constant. Therefore, at any given level of submaximal strength, EMG amplitude will vary dramatically as a function of the elbow angle since the muscle works most efficiently in terms of strength at only one optimal length. This phenomena could account for some of the variability in the magnitude of the EMG in different subjects when performing a contraction at a given submaximal tension.

Obviously, variability in EMG amplitude could also occur due to differences in the mass of the muscle involved. Further, the

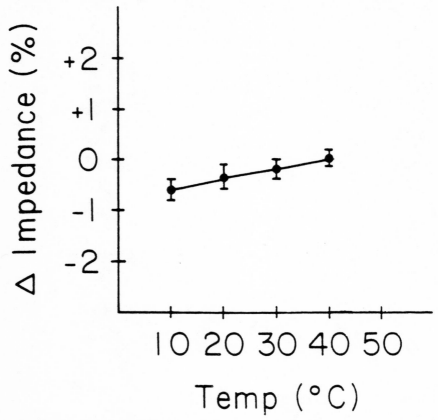

Figure 3-8.   Skin to muscle impedance as a function of bath temperature in seven subjects ± the appropriate SD. From Petrofsky and Phillips, Interrelationship Between Muscle Fatigue, Muscle Temperature, Blood Flow and the Surface EMG, © 1980 *IEEE*, 520–527, 1980. Courtesy of IEEE NAECON Record.

proximity of the electrodes to the muscle will also effect the recording of the EMG. The amplitude of motor unit action potentials is dramatically attenuated with distance from the recording electrodes. Even in muscles that are the same size, it has been shown that individuals with a thick subcutaneous fat layer have a lower EMG amplitude than individuals with a thin subcutaneous

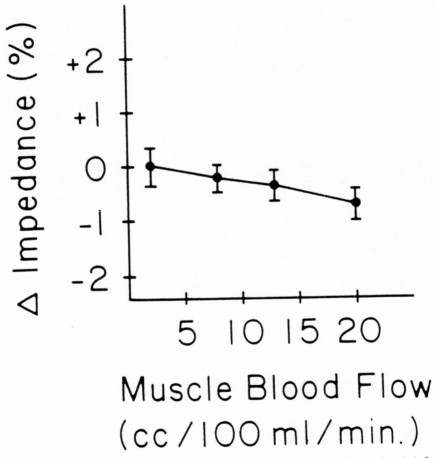

Figure 3-9.   Skin to muscle impedance in seven subjects ± the SD during brief isometric contractions (see text). From Petrofsky and Phillips, Interrelationship Between Muscle Fatigue, Muscle Temperature, Blood Flow and the Surface EMG, © 1980 *IEEE*, 520–527, 1980. Courtesy of IEEE NAECON Record.

fat layer because of the signal attentuating properties of subcutaneous fat (Lynn 1978).

II. EMG Amplitude During Fatiguing Isometric Contractions

The changes in EMG amplitude that accompany fatiguing
isometric contractions can clearly be divided into two categories.
The first of these categories is the response of the EMG
amplitude during submaximal fatiguing isometric contractions.
The second category is the response of the EMG during sustained maximal efforts. In the former type of contraction the
tension is sustained continuously at a submaximal level until,
through fatigue, the target can no longer be held. In the latter
type of exercise, an MVC is continually held, although, through
fatigue, the maximum voluntary contraction continues to drop
steadily.

When a submaximal isometric tension is sustained at the onset
of the contraction, the EMG amplitude is proportional to the
tension exerted by the muscle as described here. If that tension is

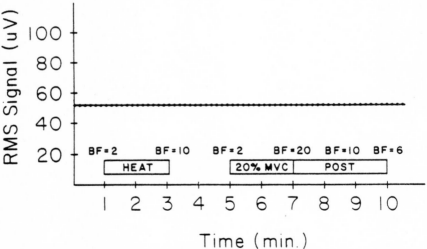

Figure 3-10.   The RMS amplitude of the signal recorded on the skin generated in muscle during passive heating of the skin and a brief
isometric contraction. From Petrofsky and Phillips, Interrelationship Between Muscle Fatigue, Muscle Temperature,
Blood Flow and the Surface EMG, © 1980 *IEEE*, 520–527,
1980. Courtesy of IEEE NAECON Record.

less than 10–15 percent MVC, then the contraction is non-fatiguing, and the EMG amplitude stays at a fairly constant level throughout the duration the contraction is held. In contrast, for sustained submaximal contractions at tensions held above 10–15 percent MVC, the EMG amplitude increases continuously throughout the contraction (Piper 1912; Cobb and Forbes 1923; Inman et al. 1952; Lippold 1952; Eason 1960; Lippold et al. 1960; Larsson et al. 1965; Moritani and DeVries 1978; Maton 1976; Petrofsky 1980; DeVries 1968; Lind and Petrofsky 1979; Petrofsky and Lind 1980). For contractions at tensions less than 70 percent MVC, the EMG amplitude increases linearly and in

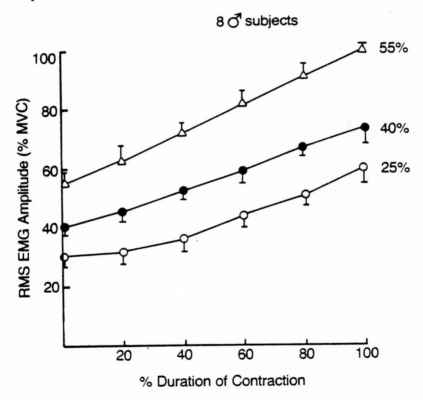

Figure 3-11.   The amplitude of the surface EMG (normalized as a percent of the EMG during an MVC in the unfatigued muscle) during fatiguing isometric contractions sustained at tensions of 25 (○), 40 (●) and 55 (△) percent MVC in four subjects ± the SD.

parallel throughout the duration of the fatiguing contractions, as shown in Figure 3-11. For contractions at tensions above 70 percent MVC, while the EMG amplitude increases linearly throughout the duration of the contraction, the EMG amplitude

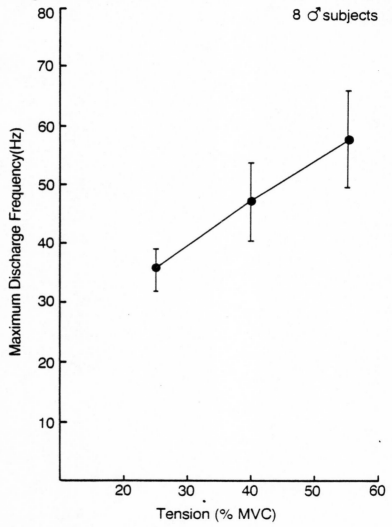

Figure 3-12. Discharge frequencies of motor units at the end of fatiguing isometric contractions in the adductor pollicis muscle of four subjects.

at the end of the fatiguing isometric contraction is always equal to that of a brief MVC. Therefore, this is in sharp contrast to the EMG amplitude at the point of fatigue for contractions at high, as compared to low, isometric tensions. For example, the EMG amplitude at the end of fatiguing isometric contractions at 25 percent MVC is only about 56 percent of the EMG amplitude during a brief MVC in the unfatigued muscle. In contrast, the EMG amplitude at the point of fatigue for contractions at 70 percent MVC is equal to that of an MVC in the fresh muscle (Lind and Petrofsky 1979). The reason that these differences occur may be linked to differences in the frequency of firing of motor units during fatiguing contractions at different isometric tensions.

During fatiguing isometric contractions at a tension of greater than 70 percent MVC, at the onset of contractions, all motor units are recruited. Therefore, the frequency of motor unit discharge is used to maintain muscle tension as the muscle fatigues. The frequency of motor unit discharge at the point of muscle fatigue in these cases is equal to approximately the same frequency found during an MVC in the unfatigued muscle, that is 60 Hz–70 Hz. In contrast, during a contraction at 25 percent MVC, initially all motor units are recruited at frequencies between 5 Hz and 15 Hz, and motor unit recruitment is used to maintain tension throughout the remaining tension. As the muscle is brought to fatigue, there is only a marginal increase in the frequency of discharge in the motor units; the final firing frequency of the alpha motor units under these conditions ranges between 30 Hz and 40 Hz. For contractions between 25 and 70 percent MVC, a proportional increase in the frequency of discharge in the motor units is seen towards the end of fatiguing contractions. Since the amplitude of the surface EMG is an algebraic summation of the frequency of motor unit discharge and the motor unit recruitment, these changes in discharge patterns are sufficient to account for lower EMG amplitude at the point of fatigue during isometric contractions at tensions less than 70 percent MVC, as shown in Figure 3-12.

Muscle temperature has little effect on the amplitude of the surface EMG during fatiguing isometric contractions over the temperature range of 28°–38° C (Petrofsky and Phillips 1980B;

Petrofsky and Lind 1980; Frauendorf et al. 1974). For example, Figure 3-13 compares the change in EMG amplitude with time during fatiguing isometric contractions at 25, 40, 55 and 70 percent MVC. Although the amplitude of the EMG varies somewhat with temperature, the pattern of response is nearly the same for isometric contractions performed at both temperatures.

In contrast to this response, relating the changes in EMG amplitude with time throughout the duration of fatiguing

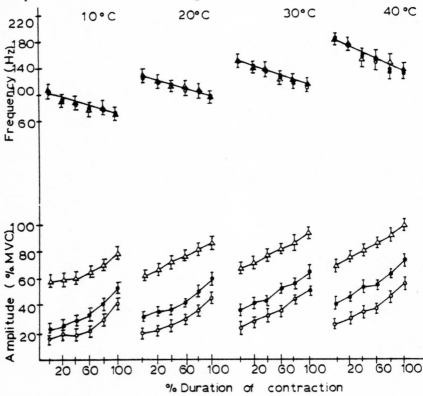

Figure 3-13.   The RMS amplitude and center frequency of the power spectra of the surface EMG during fatiguing isometric contractions at tensions of 25 (○), 40 (●), and 70 (△) percent MVC after immersion in water at 10°, 20°, 30°, and 40°C. Each point illustrates the mean of two experiments on each of ten subjects ± SD. From Petrofsky and Lind, Frequency Analysis of the Surface EMG During Sustained Isometric Exercise, *Eur J Appl Physiol*, 173–182, 1980. Courtesy of Chelsen College, University of London.

isometric contractions during sustained maximal effort, the EMG amplitude starts at the level of the MVC of the unfatigued muscle and drops almost continuously as the contraction is held. The changes in EMG amplitude and tension during sustained maximal effort were first described by Stephens and Taylor (1972). As illustrated in Figure 3-14, in the first few minutes of holding a sustained maximal effort, tension falls rapidly and in parallel with the EMG amplitude. However, after 3–5 minutes, the tension has been reduced to less than 50 percent of the original MVC and then begins to slowly fall even further (Lind and Petrofsky 1979). In contrast, the EMG amplitude begins to plateau at about 50 percent of the amplitude of the EMG for a brief MVC in the fatigued muscle (*See* Figure 4-14). Originally, Stephens and Taylor (1972) proposed that the initial stages of fatigue during a sustained maximal effort were in fact due to electrical failure of either the neuromuscular junction, or the sarcolemma, to propagate action potentials to the muscle. They proposed that the latter phase of fatigue was fatigue of the contractile components due to some type of metabolic failure. However, as was the case for sustained submaximal isometric contractions, Bigland-Ritchie and Lippold (1980) have found that

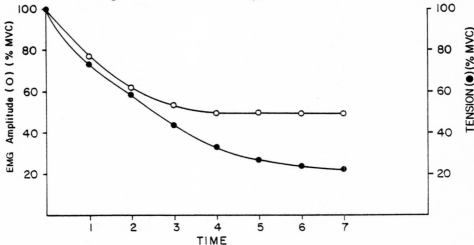

Figure 3-14.   The reduction in the EMG amplitude (o) and force (•) during a sustained maximal effort.

the rapid fall in the EMG amplitude is due to the reduction in the frequency of firing of motor units and not to a failure of transmission (Bigland-Richie, and Lippold, 1979, 1980). At the onset of a sustained maximal effort, the firing frequency of motor units averages 60 Hz–70 Hz. However, over the first 3–5 minutes of a sustained maximal effort, the frequency of discharge of the motor units falls linearly to approximately 30 Hz–40 Hz (Marsden et al. 1976; Bigland-Richie and Lippold 1979, 1980). These changes in frequency of discharge are of sufficient intensity to account for the fall in EMG amplitude observed by Stephens and Taylor (1972).

It is probable that changes in the frequency of motor unit discharge over this frequency range will have no impact on the tension developed by the muscle. In man, during fatiguing isometric contractions, and in the cat, it has been shown that the amplitude of the action potentials conducted across the sarcolemma will be reduced by no more than 5 percent during fatiguing isometric contractions (Ochs et al. 1977). Further, there is an increase in the duration of the motor unit action potentials by 30–40 percent during fatiguing static effort. The overall result, then, was that the integrated area under the muscle fiber action potentials actually increases during fatiguing isometric exercise. Fink and Luttgau (1976) showed that similar changes in the amplitude and duration of muscle fiber action potentials had no impact on the contractile characteristics of muscle. It is possible that the reduction in the frequency of motor unit discharge could reduce the tension developed by a muscle during isometric contractions and, thereby, partially account for fatigue. However, although the fresh muscle (unfatigued) requires frequencies of motor unit discharge as high as 40 Hz–50 Hz to fully tetanize the muscle, fatigued muscle tetanizes at much lower frequencies (Petrofsky and Lind 1979; Edwards et al. 1977). This appears to be due to the fact that there is a reduction in ATP turnover and actomyocin ATPase activity in muscle fatigued during isometric contractions (Edwards et al. 1975; Petrofsky, Weber, and Phillips 1980; Petrofsky, Guard and Phillips 1979; Petrofsky et al. 1980). Therefore, although the frequency of motor unit discharge is lower at the point of fatigue for contractions at tensions between 25 and 70 percent MVC, there may be no reduction in the maximum tetanic tension developed by the muscle. This same argument holds for both sustained submaximal and maximal isometric contractions.

Frequency Components of the Surface EMG During Fatiguing Isometric Contractions

Ever since Piper (1912) and later Cobb and Forbes (1923) and Denny-Brown (1924, 1926) first noticed that there was a reduction in the basic rhythm of "carrier" frequency of the EMG during powerful isometric contractions, there has been a great deal of interest in using the frequency components of the surface EMG as a diagnostic tool with which to quantify muscular fatigue, particularly during isometric exercise. However, the EMG is a very complex waveform, and visual analysis of the surface EMG has proven tedious and inadequate. Beginning in the 1950s, there has been an exponential increase in the literature examining the frequency components of the EMG that has paralleled the increase in electronic sophistication found in physiological and neurological laboratories. Beginning in the early 1950s, investigators began to use automated electronic means of analyzing the frequency components of the EMG. Some of these analysis techniques involved frequency selective amplification, zero-crossing detectors, and rapid analog differentiation of the raw EMG waveform (Fusfeld 1971, 1972; Kogi and Hakamada 1962; Ortengren 1975; Dietz and Volker 1978; Kopec et al. 1966; Moosa and Brown 1972; Stulen and DeLuca 1978; Fever and DeLuca 1976; Petrofsky 1980; Pearce and Shaw 1965). However, it was not until the early 1960s that more sophisticated digital computer analytic techniques evolved that allowed for easier assessment of the frequency components of the surface EMG. In the early 1960s using a digital computer to analyze the frequency components of the EMG, or by using filter bank frequency analyzers, it was found that during fatiguing isometric contractions there was an increase in the power in the low-frequency components of the EMG and a decrease in the relative power of the high frequency of the EMG when muscles are fatigued (Kogi and Hakamada 1962). It was, therefore, suggested that a ratio of the low- and high-frequency components of the EMG might be a useful fatigue index (Lindström et al. 1970). Typically, the ratio of power in low (30 Hz–50 Hz band) and high (300 Hz–500 Hz) frequencies has been used as a fatigue index. However, the ratio of the power components, while providing a qualitative index of the onset of fatigue, has proved to be far too unreliable to quantitate fatigue successfully.

The real breakthrough in the automatic analysis of the EMG really came in 1966 with the development of the Fast Fourier Transform (FFT) by Cooley and Tukey (1965). These mathematicians discovered a way of using a digital computer to analyze the frequency components of a complex wave-form, such as the EMG, in a few seconds of computer time. Using this technique, all of the frequency components within the audio frequency range can be analyzed quickly and efficiently. Fourier analysis of the frequency components of the EMG has become very popular in the last twenty years (Yoo et al. 1979; Viitasalo and Komi 1977; Kasser and Lehr 1979; Lloyd 1970; Lindström et al. 1970; Cenkovich and Gersten 1963; Petrofsky 1980; Petrofsky et al. 1975, 1977, 1979, 1980). A typical example of the frequency components of the EMG during a brief isometric contraction at 40 percent MVC is shown in Figure 3-15. This diagram shows an EMG recording from the flexor muscles of the forearm during a handgrip contraction. During this contraction, it can be seen that the majority of the power of the surface EMG resides in the band width of 30 Hz–70 Hz. This agrees well with the initial finding of Piper (1912) that the carrier frequency of the EMG had a basic frequency of about 60 Hz. At higher frequencies, the power of the EMG tapers off very rapidly until the effective limit of power occurs at about 300 Hz, although some power does exist above this frequency. One interesting phenomenon observed by Lindström (1970, 1977) and his colleagues was that a small dip occurred in the power of the EMG at a frequency of about 150 Hz. Analyzing the surface recording of the EMG as a transverse filter network, Lindström found that the dip was caused by the fact that power cannot be transmitted in the EMG at the frequency that occurs at the rate of conduction of action potentials across the sarcolemma of the muscle fibers.

Therefore, Lindström felt that he had an index of conduction velocity by measuring the dip frequency of the EMG. Lindström tried to use the dip frequency as an index of muscle fatigue and, in fact, found that the dip frequency decreased, as did conduc-

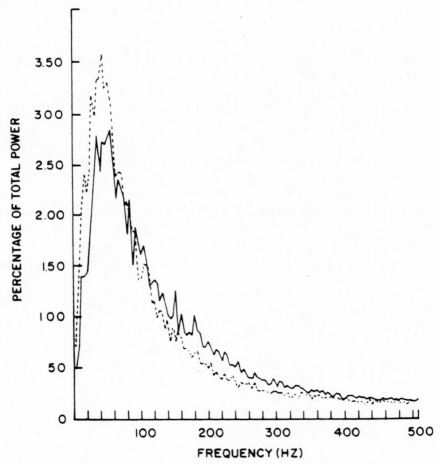

Figure 3-15.   Example of an EMG power spectrum recorded at the onset (solid line) and end (broken line) of a fatiguing isometric contraction. Power is expressed as a percentage of the total spectral power recorded at all frequencies. From Petrofsky and Lind, Frequency Analysis of the Surface EMG During Sustained Isometric Exercise, *Eur J Appl Physiol, 43*:173–182, 1980. Courtesy of Chelsen College, University of London.

tion velocity, when the muscle fatigued. However, the dip was not always seen in all individuals due to the fact that the thick subcutaneous fat layer found above muscle acts as a filter (Lynn 1978). Further, muscle movement altered the dip frequency; therefore, he found this to be an unreliable fatigue index.

In our own work (Petrofsky et al. 1975, 1978; Petrofsky 1980; Petrofsky and Lind 1980), we have found that another index of EMG frequency derived from Fourier analysis can be used as a fatigue index. Because of the complexity of the Fourier power spectra of the EMG, we tried to describe the Fourier power spectra by a single number, which would reflect the average frequency components of the EMG. In this manner, only a single measurement would be derived from each EMG sample. We chose to use the center frequency, or the centroid, of the EMG. The center frequency for a Fourier power spectra is defined as that frequency above and below that the power in the spectra is equal. Because there is some power in the frequency spectrum extending up to 300 Hz, the center frequency of the spectrum as shown in Figure 3-15 is pushed upwards from the frequency where the most power occurs. For example, in this figure, the center frequency (average frequency) of the Fourier power spectra would be about 152 Hz.

When the Fourier power spectra is measured for 1.5-second EMG samples during brief isometric contractions (less than 3 seconds), it is found that the frequency components of the EMG are not affected to any large extent by the tension exerted by the muscle. Therefore, the center frequency of the Fourier power spectra of the EMG is relatively independent of the tension exerted by the muscle as well (*See* Figure 3-16) (Petrofsky et al. 1975; Petrofsky and Lind 1980). These results in our own lab were confirmed by Viitasalo and Komi (1977) for tensions up to 70 percent MVC. However, for stronger isometric contractions, Viitasalo and Komi found that there was a small reduction in the center frequency of the surface EMG during powerful isometric contractions. In their experiments, contractions were sustained for a longer period of time. Since the contractions at 80–100 percent MVC can only be sustained for a few seconds before fatigue develops, it is probable that these investigators were looking at partially fatigued muscle and this resulted in the drop in center frequency as described next.

During fatiguing isometric contractions, center frequency drops dramatically. For example, when contractions are sustained at a tension of 40 percent MVC to fatigue in the handgrip muscles, there is a linear fall in the center frequency of the Fourier power spectra throughout the duration of a fatiguing isometric contraction (*See* Figure 3-17). Further, the reduction in center frequency during fatiguing contractions, like tension during brief isometric contractions, appears to be independent of the tension exerted by the muscle. When contractions were sustained in four male subjects by the handgrip muscles for

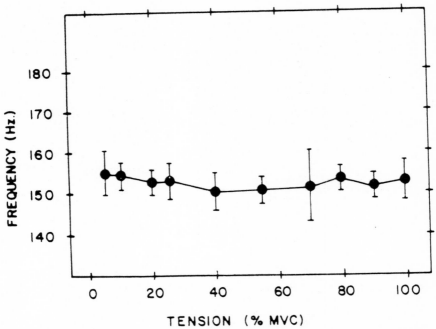

Figure 3-16.   Mean center frequencies of the EMG power spectra for EMG sampled during brief isometric contractions at tensions ranging from 5–100 percent MVC. Each point is the mean of sixteen experiments, and the bars represent ± SD. From Petrofsky and Lind, Frequency Analysis of the Surface EMG During Sustained Isometric Exercise, *Eur J Appl Physiol, 43*:173–182, 1980. Courtesy of Chelsen College, University of London.

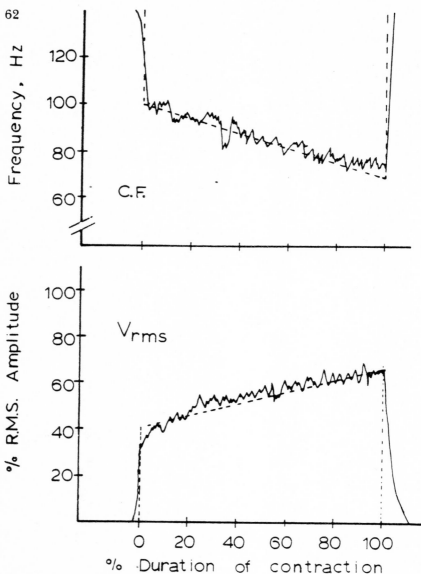

Figure 3-17. The RMS amplitude (center) and median frequency of the EMG
analysed by the filter-bank analyser during a contraction at a
tension of 40 percent MVC carried to fatigue in one subject
(solid lines). As a basis of comparison, the regression lines from a
similar analysis on a digital computer are also shown (dotted
lines). From Petrofsky, Filter Bank Analyzer for Automatic
Analysis of the EMG, *Med Biol Eng Comp*, *18*:585–590, 1980.
Copyright © 1980 IEEE.

contractions at 25, 40, 55, or 70 percent MVC, there was a linear fall in the center frequency during all contractions examined (*See* Figure 3-18). More importantly, at the point of fatigue, the center frequency always ended at the same point: approximately 117 Hz (Petrofsky 1980). Therefore, the center frequency of the EMG would appear to provide a useful fatigue index.

If the center frequency of the EMG power spectra does in fact parallel the onset of isometric fatigue, it shoud parallel the recovery from isometric contractions as well. Typically, following an isometric contraction, the muscle will recover to about 80 percent of the initial endurance in about twenty minutes; complete recovery takes in exess of twenty-four hours (Edwards et al. 1977; Lind 1959). In contrast, however, the center frequency recovers to the pre-exercise value within a few seconds following a fatiguing isometric contraction. The center frequency, as mentioned previously, appears to be related to the conduction velocity of action potentials across the sarcolemma. In animal and human experiments it has been found that the conduction velocity of action potentials will decrease during fatiguing isometric contractions (Mortimer et al. 1970; Petrofsky et al. 1979, 1980). The conduction velocity of action potential following fatiguing contractions, like the center frequency, recovers in a few seconds following a fatiguing static effort (Petrofsky et al. 1980). It would, therefore, appear that while the center frequency of the EMG power spectra is correlated with the onset of muscle fatigue, whatever phenomena causes muscle fatigue recovers at a different rate than the EMG center frequency. However, in successive isometric contractions, the center frequency of the surface EMG still ends at the same final value at the point of fatigue. Further, since this point is always about 25 percent less than the center frequency in the unfatigued muscle, by looking at the rate of decrease of EMG center frequency during a fifteen- or twenty-second sample of EMG and by knowing the end point, the center frequency may still be used as a predictive tool to predict the duration of the fatiguing isometric contractions. This can be accomplished with the following equation:

$$D = ([\,100 - (100F_{c2}/F_{c1})\,] / 24)\,100$$

where
D = % duration of the contraction
F_{c2} = Current EMG center frequency (Hz)
F_{c1} = Center frequency of the EMG during a brief
      MVC in the unfatigued muscle (Hz)

Although the center frequency of the EMG power spectra during brief isometric contractions in most people is about 150 Hz, there are several factors that may cause this figure to vary. One such factor is the position of the EMG electrodes. Since the center frequency of the EMG power spectra is affected by the

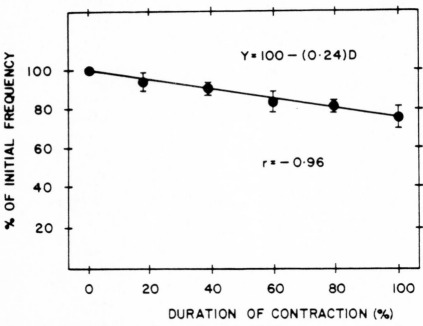

Figure 3-18.   Mean center frequencies of the EMG power spectra throughout fatiguing isometric contractions at tensions of 25, 40, 55, 70, 80 and 90 percent MVC normalized in terms of the center frequency recorded at the onset of the contraction. Each point is the mean of 96 experiments ± SD. From Petrofsky and Lind, Frequency Analysis of the Surface EMG During Sustained Isometric Exercise, *Eur J Appl Physiol, 43*:173–182, 1980. Courtesy of Chelsen College, University of London.

conduction velocity of action potentials across the sarcolemma, the orientation of the muscle fibers as well as electrode position alters the amplitude of the frequency components of the EMG (Lynn 1978; Buchthal et al. 1954, 1955). It is, therefore, very important to stabilize electrode position from day to day and from suject to subject to minimize this variation.

One factor that can dramatically influence the frequency components of the surface EMG is muscle temperature. The conduction velocity of action potentials across the sarcolemma is directly proportional to the temperature of the muscle. A change in muscle temperature from 28° to 38° C can double the conduction velocity of action potentials. A similar phenomenon occurs with the center frequency. As shown in Figure 3-19, there is a reduction in the low-frequency components and a general shift into the high-frequency region when the muscle temperature changes from 28° to 38° C during a brief isometric contraction at 40 percent MVC. The center frequency changes from 110 Hz to 152.5 Hz under these experimental conditions. Therefore, even a change of a few degrees centigrade during an experiment can alter the EMG center frequency more than that which occurs due to muscle fatigue. It is very important to stabilize muscle temperature throughout the experiment. However, since the resting muscle temperature varies so widely due to environmental and inherent influences, it is equally important to know what changes occur in the center frequency during isometric contractions at widely different muscle temperatures. Fortunately, the reduction in the center frequency of the EMG remains constant at about 25 percent during a fatiguing isometric contraction irrespective of the muscle temperature. For example, in Figure 3-13, fatiguing isometric contractions were performed at muscle temperatures between 22°-37° C. Although the center frequency was dramatically reduced when the muscle temperature was lowered, the center frequency always decreased by about 25 percent during the fatiguing isometric

Isometric Exercise and Its Clinical Implications

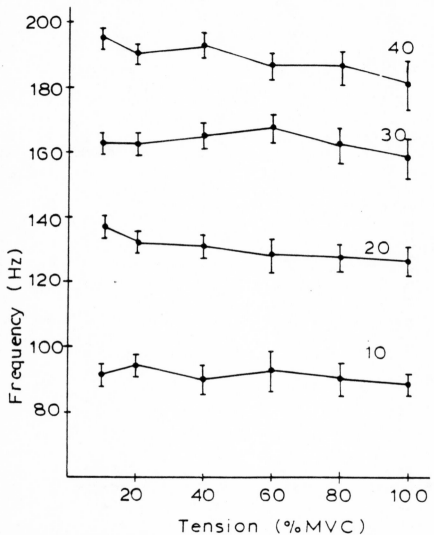

Figure 3-19. The center frequency of the EMG power spectra during brief
isometric contractions at four bath temperatures of 10°, 20°, 30°,
and 40° C. Each point illustrates the mean of two experiments
on each of ten subjects ± SD. From Petrofsky and Lind, the Influence of Temperature on the Amplitude and Frequency
Components, *Eur J Appl Physiol, 44*:189–200, 1980. Courtesy of
Springer-Verlag New York, Inc.

contractions. Therefore, the center frequency of the surface EMG may provide a good fatigue index for isometric contractions.

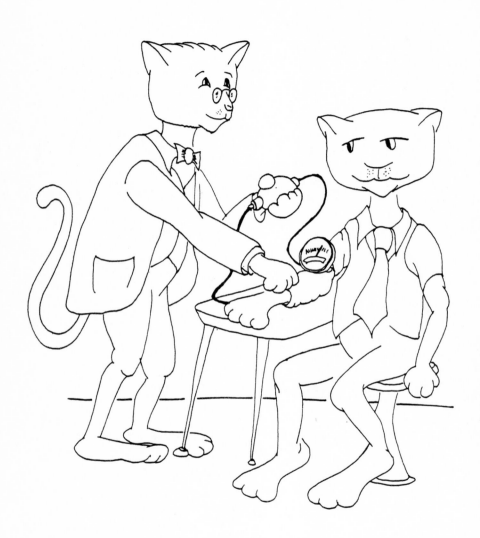

CHAPTER 4

THE CARDIORESPIRATORY RESPONSES DURING ISOMETRIC EXERCISE

BLOOD PRESSURE RESPONSE TO ISOMETRIC EXERCISE

U nlike dynamic exercise where mean blood pressure usually increases very little, Lindhard (1920) first noticed that there was a dramatic rise in both the systolic and diastolic blood pressure during fatiguing isometric contractions. This early observation, which was confirmed later by Alam and Smirk (1937, 1938) and by Asmussen and Hansen (1938), aroused a great deal of interest in the field of isometric exercise physiology. Interest in this phenomena was rekindled by Tuttle and Horvath (1957) and, in the early 1960s, in a classic series of experiments by Lind and his colleagues (Humphreys and Lind 1963; Lind et al. 1964; Staunton et al. 1964; McDonald et al. 1966; Lind and McNicol 1967; Donald et al. 1967; Lind et al. 1968; Muir and Donald 1968).

When contractions are sustained at non-fatiguing tensions (less than 15 percent MVC), the blood pressure rises in proportion to the tension exerted by the muscles. During contractions at 5 percent MVC both the systolic and diastolic blood pressure may increase by 5-10mm Hg. For contractions at 10 percent MVC the increase in blood pressure is about double this. During contractions at these tensions, once the blood pressure increases, it stays constant throughout the duration the tensions are sustained. In contrast, during contractions sustained at fatiguing tensions, there is a continuous increase in blood pressure throughout the duration of the contractions (Lind et al. 1964; Funderburk et al. 1974). The blood pressure response of a typical subject during a contraction at 40 percent MVC is shown in Figure 4-1. As can be seen in this figure, throughout the dura-

69

tion of the contration (some 2.5 minutes) both the systolic and diastolic pressures rose in parallel and continuously throughout the duration of the contractions. At the point of fatigue, the blood pressure in most subjects is typically 50 percent or more above the resting level (Petrofsky and Lind 1975). When two submaximal contractions are sustained together with two different muscle groups, the pressure response is additive (*See* Figure 4-2) (Lind and McNicol 1967). The blood pressure response is not increased if two muscles contract simultaneously (Lind and McNicol 1967). Further, this potent response is even seen in patients with advanced heart disease (*See* Chapter 7) and is only marginally reduced with as much as 16 percent blood loss (Bergenwald et al. 1977). However, there is a great deal of variation in the blood pressure response among individuals. In some subjects there is only a modest increase in the blood pressure, while in others the blood pressure at least doubles during a fatiguing isometric contraction of the handgrip muscles at a tension of 40 percent MVC. The increase in blood pressure commonly associated with this form of exertion does not appear to

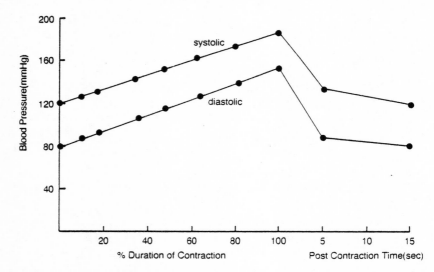

Figure 4-1.   The blood pressure recorded from a typical subject during a fatiguing isometric contraction of the handgrip muscles at a tension of 40 percent MVC.

alter the normal baroreceptor reflex (Mancia et al. 1977; Ludbrook et al. 1978). In the face of a large increase in mean blood

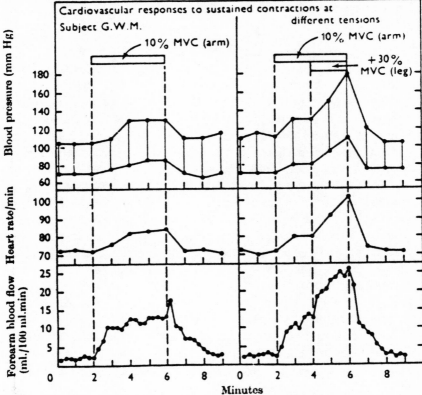

Figure 4-2.   During a handgrip at 10 percent MVC for four minutes (See left side), the forearm blood flow, blood pressure, and heart rate all rose to a steady state, which was maintained throughout the contraction. The right half of the figure shows the responses when the "test" arm repeated that contraction but, during the last two minutes of the handgrip, the leg also contracted at 30 percent MVC. The cardiovascular responses were the same when the hand gripped by itself, but, when the leg contraction at 30 percent MVC was superimposed on the forearm contraction, there was a progressive rise of blood pressure, and heart rate as well, of the blood flow through the "test" forearm. From Lind and McNicol, Circulatory Responses to Sustained Handgrip Contractions Performed During Other Exercise, Both Rhythmic and Static, *J Physiol*, 595–604, 1967. Courtesy of Journal of Physiology, London.

pressure, the baroreceptor reflex is normal; apparently the baseline pressure is simply elevated by a mechanism that is currently obscure.

Aging

Some of the variation observed in a large population of individuals in the blood pressure response associated with isometric exercise can be attributed to aging. As men and women get older, there is an increase in both the systolic and diastolic blood pressure at rest. During a fatiguing isometric contraction, there is both a greater increase in the systolic blood pressure throughout the duration of the contraction and in the rate of rise of blood pressure in older individuals, as is shown in the blood pressure recorded at the end of an isometric contraction in 183 men and women of the handgrip muscles at a tension of 40 percent MVC (*See* Figure 4-3). In women, the systolic and diastolic blood pressure is generally less than that of men in the second and third decades of life. However, by the fifth and sixth decades of life, the resting systolic and diastolic blood pressures are equal in men and women (Petrofsky and Lind 1975; Petrofsky, Burse, and Lind 1975). These were also our findings during isometric contractions. The greatest rate of rise in blood pressure during a fatiguing isometric contraction was always found in the males in the second and third decade of life. However, by the fifth and sixth decade, the increase in blood pressure thoughout the duration of a fatiguing isometric contraction was the same in both men and women. The increased rate of rise of blood pressure throughout the duration of a fatiguing isometric contraction associated with the aging process is probably attributable to arteriosclerosis associated with the aging process, reducing the compliance of the large arteries. Although aging accounts for a large degree of the variation in the blood pressure response between individuals in a large population, much of the variation in blood pressure response cannot be accounted for in terms of this variable.

Muscle Mass

Mitchell and his colleagues (Mitchell and Wildenthal 1974; Mitchell 1976; Saltin and Mitchell 1978; Mitchell 1980) and

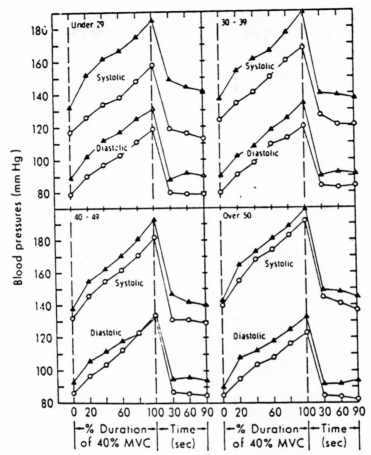

Figure 4-3.   The average blood pressures of men (▲) and women (○) in each of
the four decades are represented in the separate panels. Systolic
and diastolic blood pressures are shown before, during, and after
the fatiguing 40 percent MVC handgrip contraction. From Petrofsky, Burse, and Lind, Comparison of Physiological Responses
of Women and Men to Isometric Exercise, *J Appl Physiol,*
38:863–868, 1975. Courtesy of The American Physiological
Society.

Buck (1980) and Rowell (1976, 1978) all felt that muscle mass
may be an important variable in determining the magnitude of
the blood pressure response to isometric exercise. When an
isometric contraction is sustained to fatigue, the magnitude of

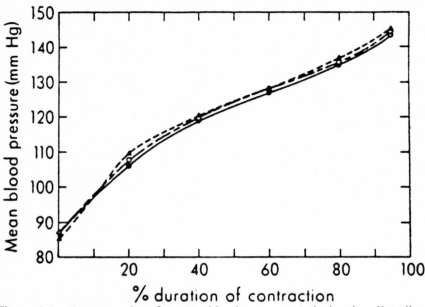

Figure 4-4.   Average values for mean blood pressures (calculated as diastolic
pressure plus one-third of pulse pressure) during sustained
handgrip contractions at 20 (○), 40 (△) and 60 percent (●) MVC.
Values shown were calculated from individual curves to permit
interpolated values at specific fractions of the duration of each
contraction; this method was chosen to permit normalization of
the findings from different tensions that yielded different absolute durations and also took account of the variable individual
duration of contractions. From Funderburk et al., Isometric
Exercise and Its Clinical Implications, *J Appl Physiol, 37*:392-401,
1974. Courtesy of The American Physiological Society.

the blood pressure response is the same, irrespective of the tension exerted by the muscle, as long as the same muscle is doing
the exercise (*See* Figure 4-4) (DeVries and Adams 1972; Funderburk et al. 1974). However, when large muscles sustain isometric
contractions for set periods of time, there appears to be a larger
blood pressure response than that which is found for small muscle groups contracting over the same time period (Mitchell 1974,
1976, 1978, 1980; McCloskey and Streatfield 1975). Further-
more, in these studies, isometric contractions were never sustained to fatigue. But different muscle groups in various parts of
the body have different muscle temperatures. Typically, larger

muscle groups such as those studied by Mitchell and his colleagues are located closer to the core than are smaller muscle groups such as those that control the handgrip. Therefore, these muscle groups have a much higher muscle temperature (Barcroft and Millen 1939; Barcroft and Edhohm 1943; Clarke, Hellon, and Lind 1958). As described in Chapter 2 on *Isometric Strength and Endurance*, these muscles have a lower isometric endurance than the small muscle groups of the forearm. For this reason, the larger muscle groups may have been brought closer to fatigue than was the case for the small muscle groups, and, therefore, it is not surprising that the rise in blood pressure was higher during the contraction of large muscle groups. The exact relationship between muscle mass and the cardiovascular responses to isometric exercise is yet to be determined.

Neural Pathways

The mechanism of the blood pressure response to isometric exercise has been the subject of a great deal of interest, particularly in the last thirty years, although the idea of a chemical stimulus arising from skeletal muscle was first proposed by Zuntz and Geppart (1888). The response appears to originate mainly from afferent nerve fibers in active skeletal muscle causing a reflex increase in sympathetic tone to the splanchnic bed; Sympathetic blocking agents abolish the pressor response (Freyscuss 1970; Martin et al. 1974). This can be seen quite readily in the laboratory with a very simple experiment. If an occlusion cuff is placed on the upper arm and it is inflated to above 250 mm Hg, the circulation to the contracting muscle will be occluded throughout the duration of contractions of the handgrip muscles. During this contraction the blood pressure rises in the same manner and to the same degree as occurs with the circulation to the muscle free (Lind et al. 1964; Staunton et al. 1964). Therefore, the release of a chemical vasoconstrictor substance from the muscle, which enters the central circulation, can be eliminated as the causative agent for the blood pressure response to isometric exercise. If the contraction is released, and the blood pressure cuff remains inflated, the blood pressure remains elevated at nearly the same level as occurred at the end of the fatiguing isometric contraction, as long as the blood pressure cuff is inflated (*See* Figure 4-5) (Staunton et al. 1964). If the blood pressure cuff is released, the blood pressure rapidly returns to the pre-exercise values. This early experiment provided definitive evidence that the afferent arm of the blood pressure response was nervous in origin arising from the active skeletal muscle. Further, Lind and his colleagues (1968) found that a patient with unilateral syringomyelia (a disease effecting muscle afferants) caused the blood pressure response during isometric exercise to be abolished on the affected side but allowed a normal blood pressure response to occur on the unaffected side of

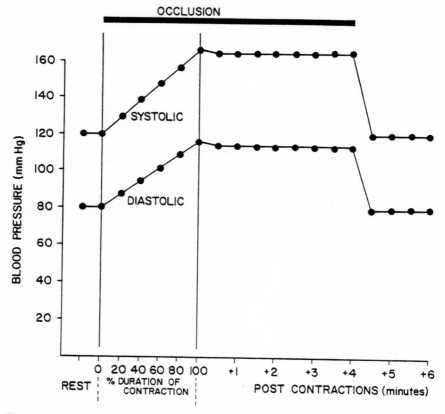

Figure 4-5.   The blood pressure response that occurs during and after an isometric contraction at 40 percent MVC of the handgrip muscles, with the circulation free (●) and occluded (○).

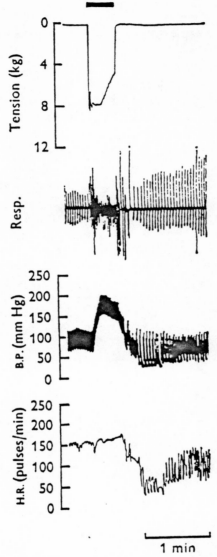

Figure 4-6. *Decerebrate Cat.* Records (from above, downwards) of tension developed by triceps surae, respiration (Resp.), arterial blood pressure (B.P.) and heart rate (H.R.). At signal, tetanic contraction of
the right hind-limb muscles elicited by stimulating peripheral cut
ends of ventral roots (L6–S1, at 0.3v and 50 Hz. Both common
carotid arteries tied. From Coote et al., The Reflex Nature of the
Pressor Response to Muscular Isometric Exercise, *J Physiol,*
215:789–804, 1971. Courtesy of Journal of Physiology.

the body. These experiment provided additional evidence for the peripheral nervous origin of the blood pressure response during isometric exercise.

Definitive evidence as to the exact nervous pathways involved was not discovered until some five years later. In separate experiments, Coote, Hilton, and Perez-Gonzales (1971) and McClosky and Mitchell (1972) all found that if one of the hindlimb muscles in the cat was fixed and stimulated through the ventral roots of the spinal cord, so that it could contract isometrically, there was an increase in both systolic and diastolic blood pressure during these contractions (*See* Figure 4-6). Since anodal block of the type III and IV sensory fibers or destruction of the whole dorsal roots that carry the afferent sensory information from these muscles (L6, L7, S1) abolishes the blood pressure response, the blood pressure response to isometric exercise is considered to be mediated through small, unmyelinated sensory

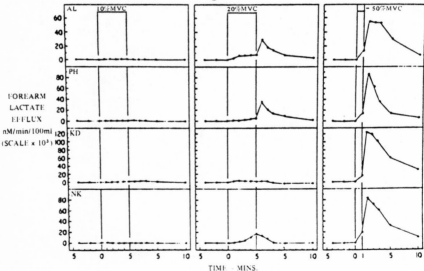

Figure 4-7.   Forearm lactate ion efflux before, during, and after sustained handgrip contractions (10, 20, and 50% MVC) in four normal subjects. These results are calculated from deep forearm venous concentrations and forearm blood flow determined in separate experiments. From Lind et al., *Physical Activity in Health and Disease*, pp. 38–63, 1966. Courtesy of Williams and Wilkins, Baltimore.

nerve afferant fibers. Skeletal muscle is innervated extensively by type III and IV sensory fibers (Ranson and Davenport 1931; Clement et al. 1973; Hnik et al. 1969; Freund et al. 1979; Kumazama and Mizumura 1977). The ends of these nerves for the most part can be seen as naked nerve endings interweaved throughout the interstitial space in skeletal muscle. The purpose of the majority of these nerve fibers is not known. It has been suggested by Lind et al. (1964) and Hnik et al. (1969) that a metabolite released from isometrically contracting skeletal muscle stimulates these nerve endings and initiates the blood pressure response to isometric exercise. In both man and in the cat the blood pressure rises linearly throughout the duration of fatiguing isometric contractions. Following the contractions, the blood pressure returns to the control values within a few seconds. Therefore, it is likely that the metabolite that mediates the blood pressure response must accumulate in concentrations and in a time course that parallels the blood pressure response. In-

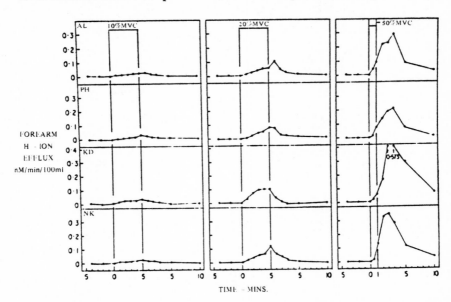

Figure 4-8. Forearm H^+ efflux before, during, and after sustained handgrip contractions in four normal subjects (See text to Figure 4-6.) From Lind et al., *Physical Activity in Health and Disease*, pp. 38–63, 1966. Courtesy of Williams and Wilkins, Baltimore.

terstitial oxygen content, lactic acid concentration in the muscle, muscle hydrogen ion content, muscle PCO_2, and most other metabolites do not fit into this category because they remain in high concentration within skeletal muscle for some time following a fatiguing isometric contraction. The only metabolite that parallels these changes in the blood pressure is potassium (Lind et al. 1964), as shown in Figures 4-6, 4-7, 4-8, and 4-9.

During the contraction of skeletal muscle (either dynamic or static), potassium is lost from the intracellular space to the interstitial space and into the blood. The increase in venous outflow of potassium during static exercise mirrors the changes in blood pressure, both in magnitude and time course, during and following isometric contractions. Potassium, therefore, was proposed as a candidate for mediating the blood pressure response to isometric exercise. No definitive studies localizing specific potassium receptors in skeletal muscle have been accomplished. However, naked nerve endings are extremely sensitive to the concentration of extracellular potassium.

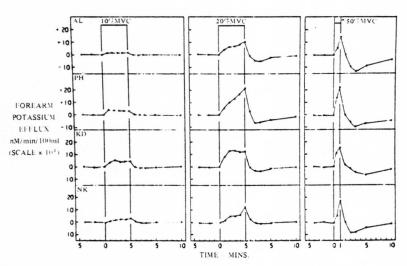

Figure 4-9.   Forearm potassium efflux before, during, and after sustained handgrip contractions in four normal subjects (See text to Figure 4-6.) From Lind et al., *Physical Activity in Health and Disease,* pp. 38–63, 1966. Courtesy of Williams and Wilkins, Baltimore.

Role of Fiber Type

In man, fiber composition of muscle has been found to be correlated to the blood pressure response during isometric exercise (Frisk-Holmberg et al. 1979, 1980). Further, in the cat, it also appears that the fiber composition of the muscles has an important role in determining the blood pressure response during isometric exercise. By sequentially stimulating the ventral roots of the spinal cord innervating the lower-limb muscles of the cat, it is possible to elicit the same increase in blood pressure as that which occurs in man during isometric exercise (*See* Figure 4-10) (Petrofsky, Phillips, and Lind 1980). Contraction of the medial gastrocnemius muscle, a fast-twitch muscle, elicits a powerful pressor response (*See* Figure 4-11). Stimulation of the ventral roots innervating the soleus muscle in the cat does not, however, cause a significant increase in blood pressure (Petrofsky and Lind, Petrofsky et al. 1981). Pharmacological blockage of the fast-twitch motor units in the medial gastrocnemius muscle

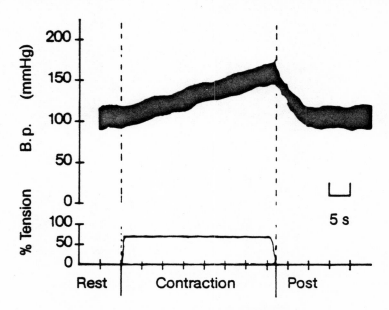

Figure 4-10. A typical tracing of the blood pressure and tension developed in a cat during contraction of the medial gastrocnemius muscle.

blocks the pressor response in this muscle (*See* Figure 4-12). During a contraction of the soleus muscle or the slow-twitch motor units in the medial gastrocnemius muscle, the concentration of potassium in the venous effluent of these muscles increases by only about one milliequivalent. In contrast, during contraction of the entire medial gastrocnemius muscle, the potassium concentration in the venous effluent blood increased by over 5 meq per liter (*See* Figure 4-13). This phenomena may explain some of the differences in the blood pressure response found between individuals in man, since the composition of muscles varies greatly due to genetic makeup and physical training (Dubowitz and Brooke 1974).

Central Component of the Blood Pressure Response

Although most of the blood pressure response is certainly linked to peripheral receptors, a "central component" of the blood pressure response has been demonstrated. Corbett et al.

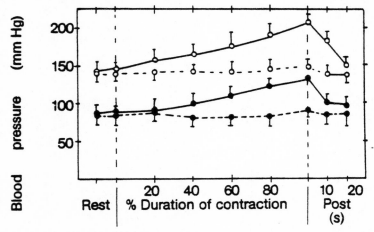

Figure 4-11.   The systolic (open symbols) and diastolic (closed symbols) blood pressures ($\pm$ the SD) recorded at the onset and at 20, 40, 60, 80, and 100 percent of the duration and 10 and 20(s) after fatiguing isometric contractions in the medial gastrocnemius (solid lines) and soleus (broken lines) muscle of the cat. Each point illustrates the average of four experiments on four different cats $\pm$ the SD. From Petrofsky et al., Blood Flow And Metabolic Products During Fatiguing Isometric Contractions, *J Appl Physiol, 50*:32–37, 1981. Courtesy of The American Physiological Society.

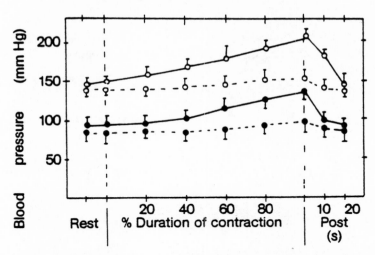

Figure 4-12. The systolic (open symbols) and diastolic (closed symbols) blood pressures recorded at the onset and at 20, 40, 60, 80, and 100 percent of the duration and 10 and 20(s) after fatiguing isometric contractions of the medial gastrocnemius muscles of the cat after administration of curare (solid lines) and decamethonium (broken lines) (see text). Each point illustrates the average of four experiments on four different cats ± the SD. From Petrofsky et al., Blood Flow and Metabolic Products During Fatiguing Isometric Contractions, *J Appl Physiol, 50*:32–37, 1981. Courtesy of The American Physiological Society.

(1970) demonstrated a blood pressure response during isometric exercise in tetraplegic patients by having them simply imagining that they were sustaining an isometric contraction. Recently, Hobbs, Rowell, and Smith (1980) have demonstrated that the blood pressure response during light isometric contractions in a baboon could be altered by varying the number of active motor units involved in a contraction by partial curarization. As the number of inactive motor units was increased to maintain a set tension, the blood pressure increased proportionally.

THE HEART RATE RESPONSE DURING ISOMETRIC EXERCISE

Unlike the blood pressure response which occurs during isometric exercise, the heart rate response during isometric exercise is much more modest. During dynamic exercise, for example, the heart rate at the end of maximal work averages about 180 beats per minute in a young individual (Astrand and Rodahl 1970). In contrast, the heart rate during isometric contractions rarely exceeds 120 beats per minute (Tuttle and Horvath 1957; Lind et al. 1964; Petrofsky, Burse, and Lind 1975; Petrofsky and Lind 1975). As reported for dynamic exercise (Simonson 1970), the maximum heart rate at the end of a fatiguing static contraction is inversely related to the age of the subject (*See* Figure 4-14). During isometric contractions at tensions that are not fatiguing, there is a small increase in heart rate

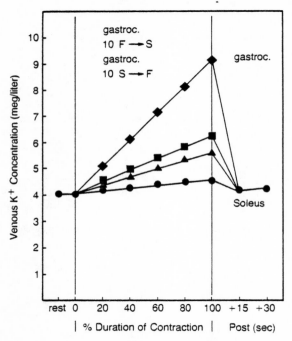

Figure 4-13.   Concentration of K$^+$ in venous effluent of: soleus muscle contracting at tensions of 40 and 70 percent of initial strength (●); medial gastrocnemius during contractions of 25, 40 and 70 percent of initial strength at all tensions and both temperatures (○); medial gastrocnemius during 10 percent contractions with recruitment from the fastest to slowest (■) rather than slowest to fastest (▲) motor units. From Petrofsky et al., Blood Flow and Metabolic Products During Fatiguing Isometric Contractions, *J Appl Physiol, 50*:32–37, 1981.

and it is maintained steadily throughout the duration of the non-fatiguing contractions (Lind et al. 1964). During a contraction, for example, at 10 percent MVC, the heart rate may increase by about 5 beats per minute and remain at this level throughout the duration of the contraction. In contrast, when a contraction is sustained at a fatiguing isometric tension, the heart rate increases steadily throughout the duration of the contraction to a final value of about 120 beats per minute in the average subject. However, the heart rate response to isometric

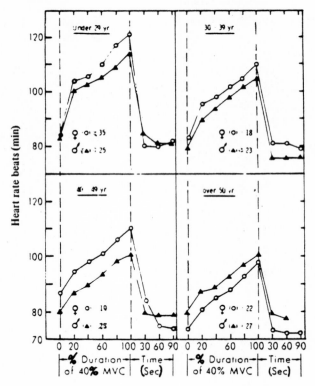

Figure 4-14. Each panel shows the average heart rates for men (▲) and women (○) in the four decades. Values are shown at rest and during and after the fatiguing 40 percent MVC contraction. From Petrofsky, Burse, and Lind, Comparison of Physiological Responses of Women and Men to Isometric Exercise, *J Appl Physiol, 38*:863–868, 1975. Courtesy of The American Physiological Society.

exercise differs in a number of ways from that of the blood pressure.

Mechanism of the Heart Rate Response

Funderburk et al. (1974), Mitchell et al. (1981), and Petrofsky et al. (1981) found that the heart rate response was related to the tension exerted by the muscle during isometric contractions. When subjects sustained isometric contractions with their handgrip muscles at tensions of 25, 40, 55, and 70 percent MVC to fatigue they found that the heart rate at the end of the fatiguing isometric contractions was directly proportional to the tension developed by the muscles (*See* Figure 4-15). Freyschuss (1970) and others (Carroll et al. 1979) found that subjects could develop a heart rate response to isometric contractions just by thinking of the contraction rather than actually doing it. She, therefore, said that the heart rate response during isometric exercise was controlled by irradiation from the central nervous system (central component). Although the experiments by Funderburk et al. seem to show proprioceptive afferents involved in the heart rate response, the difference in the heart rate at the end of the fatiguing contractions could simply be due to a different level of central effort. Further evidence of a central component is seen in that although occulsion of the circulation to a contracting muscle allows the blood pressure to remain elevated following an isometric contraction, the heart rate rapidly returns to the control value during the period when the circulation to the muscle is occluded (Staunton et al. 1964; Rowell 1976; Freund et al. 1978, 1979). Further, in the patient with unilateral syringomyelia studied by Lind and his colleagues (1968), although the blood pressure response was absent on the effected side (the side of the body with damaged muscle afferents), a heart rate response was still present. In experiments involving electrical stimulation of cat skeletal muscle, Coote, Hilton, and Perez-Gonzales (1971) and McClosky and Mitchell (1972) found a very modest change in heart rate or none at all during the isometric contractions induced by electrical stimulation of the ventral roots innervating the hind-limb muscles of the cat, whereas blood pressure increased dramatically. Finally, Petrofsky, Burse, and Lind (1981)

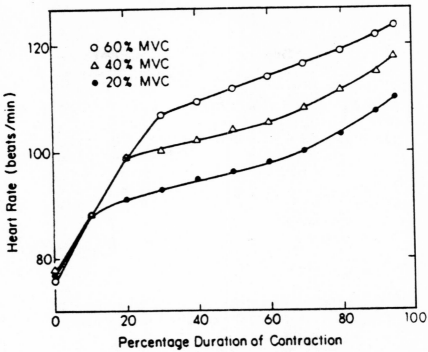

Figure 4-15.   The average heart rates during sustained handgrip contractions at 20 (●), 40 (△), and 60 (○) percent MVC. Values shown were obtained by interpolation on normalized curves obtained for heart rates in the same way as described for mean blood pressures in the legend for Figure 4-4. From Funderburk et al., the Development of and Recovery from Muscular Fatigue Induced by Static Effort at Different Tensions. *J Appl Physiol, 37*:392, 1974. Courtesy of The American Physiological Society.

found that cold-induced paralysis of skeletal muscle will block the blood pressure response during isometric exercise but have little effect on the heart rate response to isometric exercise. The evidence seems overwhelming that there is a large central component in the heart rate response to isometric exercise.

Unlike the heart rate response during dynamic exercise, Freyscuss (1970) found that the heart rate response to isometric exercise is mediated entirely through a withdrawal of vagal tone. This is a sharp contrast to the blood pressure response which is mediated by a splanchnic sympathetic vasoconstriction.

Ventilation

Oxygen uptake during isometric exercise increases modestly (*See* Figure 4-16). However, ventilation increases markedly (*See* Figure 4-17). As a result, there is a marked hyperventilation (*See* Figure 4-18) (Wiley and Lind 1971; Myrre and Andersen 1971). Like the heart rate, the ventilation returns promptly to resting levels after a contraction and in the presence of circulatory occlusion (*See* Figure 4-19). But unlike both the heart rate and the blood pressure, which increase steadily throughout an isometric contraction, there is little change in the ventilation and ventilatory equivalent until about halfway through the contraction. However, ventilation, like the blood pressure, can be increased by electrical stimulation of the ventral roots innervating skeletal muscle (Kao and Ray 1954; McCloskey and Mitchell 1972;

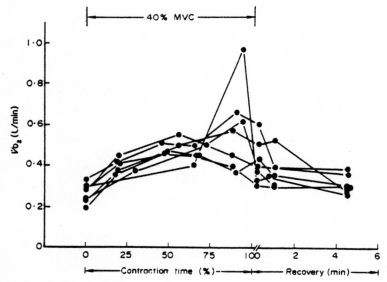

Figure 4-16.   Oxygen uptake changes during 40 percent static handgrip contractions and five minutes of recovery (seven subjects). Values for rest are the average of two 1-minute samples, taken during the third and fourth minutes of a 5-minute rest period preceding the contraction and are plotted at zero contraction time. From Wiley and Lind, Respiratory Responses to Sustained Static Muscular Contractions in Humans, *Clin Sci, 40*:221–234, 1971. Courtesy of Biochemical Society.

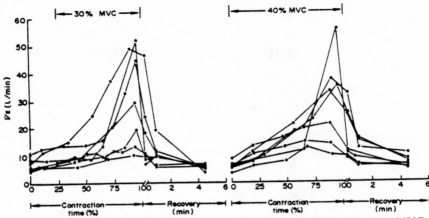

Figure 4-17. Minute ventilation changes during both 30 and 40 percent MVC handgrip contractions by seven subjects. Rest values are plotted at zero contraction time, as shown in Figure 4-16. From Wiley and Lind (1971). *Clin Sci, 40*:221–234. Reprinted with permission.

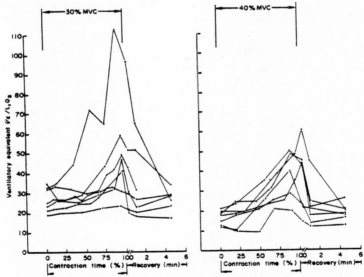

Figure 4-18. Ventilatory equivalent during 30 and 40 percent MVC handgrip contractions by seven subjects. Rest values are plotted at zero contraction time, as described in Figure 4-16. From Wiley and Lind, Respiratory Responses to Sustained Static Muscular Contraction in Humans, *Clin Sci, 40*:221–234, 1971. Courtesy of Biochemical Society.

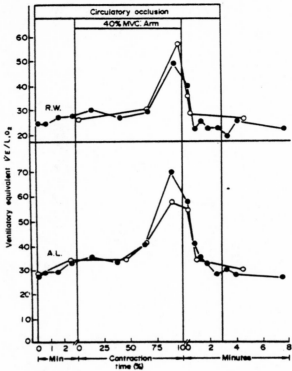

Figure 4-19.   Ventilatory equivalent from three subjects during 40 percent
MVC arm contractions with (●), and without (○), complete circulatory occlusion of the involved arm beginning a few seconds
before the release of grip and continuing for a five -minute
period (occlusion.) Rest values are plotted at zero contraction
time, as described in Figure 4-16. From Wiley and Lind, Respiratory Responses to Sustained Static Muscular Contractions
in Humans, *Clin Sci, 40*:221–234, 1971. Courtesy of Biochemical Society.

Mitchell et al. 1977) or vibration of muscle (Leitner and Dejours
1971). These responses are probably also mediated by C fibers
(Kalia et al. 1972; Mitchell et al. 1977). It seems possible that the
mechanism responsible for the changes of ventilation may be
different from those for the responses of both the blood pressure and the heart rate.

CARDIAC OUTPUT AND BLOOD
FLOW DURING ISOMETRIC CONTRACTIONS

Cardiac output increases modestly during isometric contractions. From a resting cardiac output of about five liters per minute, cardiac output usually only increases to about eight liters per minute during a fatiguing isometric contraction in most individuals (Simonson and Lind 1971; Amende et al. 1972; Miltiadis et al. 1974; Crawford et al. 1979; Crayton et al. 1979; Paulsen et al. 1979). Further, there is some evidence that as individuals grow older, cardiac output increases even less during fatiguing isometric contractions. Here, cardiac output may only increase by a liter per minute or so. Therefore, in the face of a modest increase in heart rate and cardiac output, the increase in blood pressure must be mediated by an increase in sympathetic tone. Studies in both animal and human experiments indicate that there is an increase in sympathetic tone in the splanchnic vasculature, thereby increasing peripheral resistance (Lind et al. 1964; Crayton et al. 1979). The increase in splanchnic resistance is so potent that in individuals where the increase in heart rate has been blocked due to either pharmacological intervention, blood loss, or vagotomy of the heart, the increase in blood pressure still occurs (Freyscuss 1970; Bergenwald et al. 1977; Savin et al. 1980). In the normal heart, the left ventrical maintains a constant size and displays a small fall in the peak velocity of circumferential fiber shortening (Paulsen et al. 1979; Crawford et al. 1979; Miltiadis et al. 1974; Amende et al. 1972; Bodenheimer et al. 1979). With no significant change in ejection fraction, stroke volume, or left ventricular end-diastolic pressure during this type of exertion, the increase in cardiac output apparently is due to the increase in the heart rate associated with this form of exertion (Lind et al. 1964; Simonson and Lind 1971).

The increase in blood pressure and cardiac output during isometric contractions appears to be used to maintain perfusion of the muscle during the contractions. Unlike dynamic exercise (where the muscle contracts and relaxes rhythmically, allowing a large flow of blood through the muscle during the relaxation phase), sustained isometric contractions keep intramuscular pressure high throughout the duration of the contractions. Although intramuscular pressure during isometric contractions has only been measured on a few occasions, the results of these experiments would seem to indicate that intramuscular pressure is quite high during isometric contractions, with pressure measurements in various studies ranging between 400 and 1200 mm Hg during an MVC (Edwards et al. 1972; Hill 1948; Mazzella 1954; Sylvest and Hvid 1959; Reis and Wooten 1970). Since the systolic blood pressure is considerably below this pressure, the effect on blood flow is obvious.

During submaximal isometric contractions at tensions that are non-fatiguing, blood flow increases in proportion to the tension

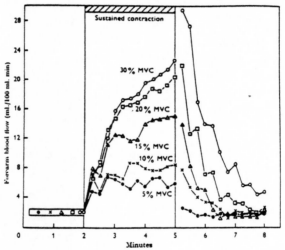

Figure 4-20.   Forearm blood flows before, during, and after a three-minute contraction at tensions from 5–30 percent MVC. At 5 and 10 percent MVC (contractions that can be held for a very long time) the blood flow reached a steady state during the contraction but afterwards fell at once. In contrast, at 20 and 30 percent MVC (a tension that quickly results in fatigue), the flows increased continuously throughout the contraction and rose after the contraction before returning to control values. At 15 percent MVC the pattern of response was intermediate — the flows did not reach a steady state during the contraction but fell immediately when the contraction ended. From Lind and McNicol, Circulatory Responses to Sustained Handgrip Contractions Performed During Other Exercise, Both Rhythmic and Static, *J Physiol,* *192*:595–604, 1967. Courtesy of Journal of Physiology.

exerted by the muscles. Like blood pressure and heart rate, the blood flow stays at a constant value throughout the duration of the non-fatiguing contractions (*See* Figure 4-20). However, during contractions at fatiguing tensions, the blood flow response is related to the tension exerted by the muscle. For example, during a contraction at 30 percent MVC, blood flow rises immediately at the onset of the contraction and continually in-

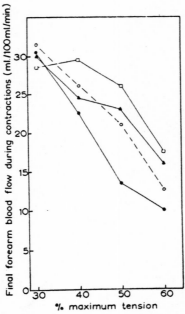

Figure 4-21.   The blood flow through the forearm in four subjects during sustained handgrip contractions held to fatigue at tensions from 30–60 percent MVC. The values shown were measured just before the end of the contractions when the blood pressure was comparable at all tensions. Blood flow could not be accurately and continuously measured at tensions of 70 percent MVC and above, because of arm movements. However, some flows were measured when the tension was 70 percent MVC; they were all small. The intramuscular pressure caused by the contracting fibers did not completely occlude the blood flow through the muscles until the tension exceeded 70 percent MVC. From Lind, McNichol and Donald, *Physical Activity in Health and Disease,* pp. 38–63, 1966. Courtesy of Williams and Wilkins, Baltimore.

creases throughout the duration of the contraction. As the contraction is terminated, blood flow increases slightly above the level found at the end of the contraction and a post-exercise hyperemia follows, lasting some 12-15 minutes (Lind et al.

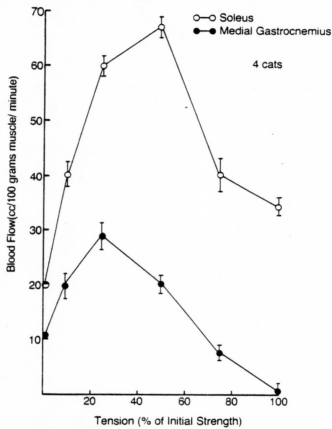

Figure 4-22.   The blood flow in the soleus and medial gastrocnemius muscles at rest (0% duration) during fatiguing and non-fatiguing isometric contractions and during a twelve-minute recovery period (post) following the exercise. Each point shows the mean of 6 cats ± the SD. The time during the contractions has been normalized in terms of the length of the contractions (% duration). From Petrofsky et al., Blood Flow and Metabolic Products During Fatiguing Isometric Contractions in Fast and Slow Skeletal Muscles in the Cat, *J Appl Physiol, 50*:493–592, 1981. Courtesy of The American Physiological Society.

1964). For contractions at 50 percent MVC, although blood flow increases at the onset of the contraction, the blood flow here is less than that recorded during a contraction of 25 percent MVC. As the contraction is sustained, the blood flow increases slightly throughout the duration of the contractions followed by a very large post-exercise hyperemia when the contraction is over, as shown in Figure 4-20. For contractions above 70 percent MVC, blood flow appears to be totally occluded by the contraction presumably due to high intramuscular pressure (*See* Figure 4-21). But the blood flow response to isometric exercise differs dramatically in different muscles in the body. In the calf muscles, for example, Barcroft and Millen (1939) and Edwards et al. (1975) found that the blood flow was totally occluded during isometric contractions at a tension greater than 30 percent MVC. They felt that the differences in the occlusion of the blood supply to the leg as opposed to the forearm muscles was not due to differences in the intramuscular pressure. They felt that for the calf muscles, the arteries, which supply blood to the muscles, were nipped off due to movement of the facial layers over the

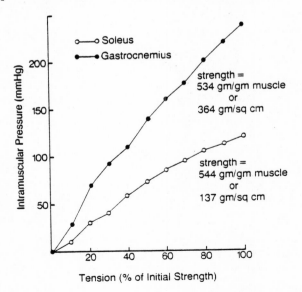

Figure 4-23. The intramuscular pressure in the soleus to medial gastrocnemius muscle of the cat during isometric contractions.

muscle during isometric contractions. In contrast, for muscles such as the handgrip it is felt that the limiting factor is that increased intramuscular pressure collapses the small arterials (Grey et al. 1967). Fiber composition of the muscles also appears to play a role in the relationship of muscle blood flow and tension during fatiguing isometric contractions. Slow-twitch muscle has been shown to have about twice the resting blood flow and twice the capillary density as is found with fast-twitch muscle (Reis and Wooten 1970; Close 1972; Folkov and Hudlichka 1967). These basic differences in the structure and organization of fast and slow muscle cause large differences in the blood flow through the muscles during the isometric contraction. In the cat, for example, the blood flow to the soleus — a slow-twitch muscle — is observed during isometric contractions, it was found that even during contractions at 100 percent of the muscle's strength for this muscle, there is still blood flow through the muscle far in excess of the resting value (*See* Figure 4-22). In contrast, in the medial gastrocnemius muscle the blood flow through the muscle was occluded during contractions above about 50 percent of the muscle's strength. These changes in blood flow during isometric contractions are paralleled by changes in intramuscular pressure in these two muscles. As shown in Figure 4-23, the intramuscular pressure at any given tension relative to the muscles maximum strength in the medial gastrocnemius muscle is always at least double that in the soleus muscle. Since the force generated per cross-sectional area of the two muscles is not dramatically different (Petrofsky et al. 1979), it must be concluded that a large part of the differences in both intramuscular pressure and blood flow must be due to the anatomical arrangement of the muscle fibers.

The mechanism controlling blood flow during and following isometric exercise has remained obsure and still remains the subject of heated controversy. Principally, the blood flow to skeletal muscle during and following exercise can be controlled by one of three means: *metabolic control,* due to the release of metabolites from the contracting muscle; *myogenic control,* due to the increased intramuscular pressure during isometric contractions; and *neurogenic control* arising from the sympathetic nervous system. Evidence exists that all three mechanisms can be involved to some extent in the control of blood flow during isometric contractions. The predominate mechanism controlling blood flow appears to be metabolic in nature. The reactive hyperemia which follows isometric exercise is not affected by sympathectomy or somatic denervation (Barcroft 1972). However, the mechanism of the reactive hyperemia which follows isometric exercise is not fully understood. A number of different factors that might be responsible have been identified. These include hypoxia, metabolites released from the muscle, and a myogenic response due to the pressure applied to the arterials during the contraction of the muscle. Arterial wall hypoxia may cause the initial dilatation of the arterials, but since the recovery of flow does not parallel the recovery of hypoxia, the role of hypoxia in sustaining the hyperemia is unlikely (Mohrman et al. 1973; Barcroft 1972). Potassium is a potent vasodilator substance (Mohrman and Sparks 1974), but its concentration in the venous blood is normal throughout the reactive hyperemia (Lind et al. 1964). Adenosine is also a potent dilator (Bockman et al. 1976) as is ATP (Forrester and Lind 1972), but their time course might also not match that of the hyperemia. Venous pH and pCO_2 are also dilators, but their time course does not match the hyperemia (Haddy and Scott 1975). Some part of the vasodilatation has been shown to be caused by a myogenic mechanism (Mohrman and Sparks 1974) but much of the hyperemia remains unexplained.

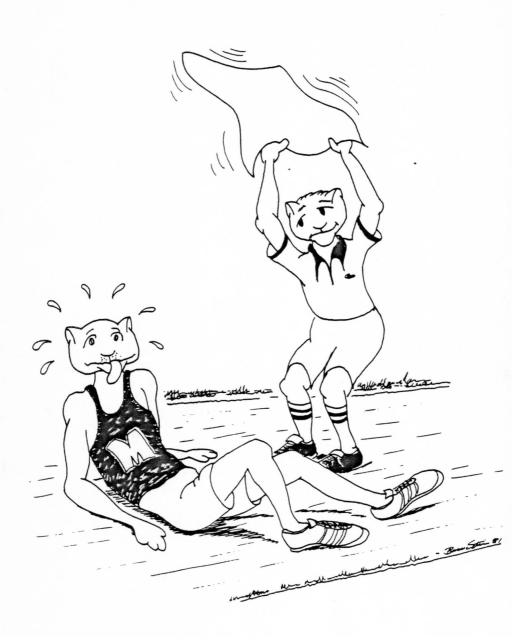

CHAPTER 5

THE ORIGIN OF MUSCLE FATIGUE DURING ISOMETRIC EXERCISE

The origin of the fatigue that accompanies isometric exercise has been very controversial in the last fifty years. Evidence exists that fatigue occurs either in the central nervous system, at the neuromuscular junction, in the propagation of action potentials across the sarcolemma, or in the contractile components of the muscle itself. Although clear evidence exists from various studies that the origin of muscle fatigue arises in one or more of the structures mentioned above, because of the diverse experimental techniques and animals used in these experiments, the results are often hard to evaluate in terms of isometric fatigue in man. It will be the purpose of this chapter to summarize the studies that have been done in order to identify the location of muscle fatigue. From these data, a potential site of muscle fatigue is proposed.

MUSCLE METABOLISM DURING ISOMETRIC CONTRACTIONS

The changes in muscle metabolism that occur during isometric exercise are much less pronounced than those that occur during dynamic exercise. When Karlsson et al. (1975) studied the changes in ATP, PC, glycogen, and lactic acid, which were found to occur in human quadriceps muscle during fatiguing isometric contractions, they found that when contractions were sustained at a tension between 30 and 50 percent MVC the reduction in ATP was by no means total (about a 20% reduction was found from the beginning to the end of the contraction), and there was still a substantial concentration of both ATP and PC present at the time of fatigue. Further, the glycogen depletion

99

patterns during the fatiguing isometric contractions at this tension showed that only about 5–10 percent of the glycogen available to the muscle was utilized during the contractions. For contractions at higher (80% MVC) and lower (20% MVC) tensions, the ATP and PC concentrations were even greater, while glycogen depletion and lactate production were even less at the point of isometric fatigue. This is in sharp contrast to dynamic exercise where glycogen depletion patterns show glycogen utilization to be almost complete at the point of fatigue during many types of dynamic exercise (Pernow and Saltin 1971). Even with a series of sustained isometric contractions, Karlsson et al. (1975) were not able to find a large reduction in the concentration of muscle glycogen. Further, for isometric tensions sustained at a tension of 20 percent MVC, glycogen utilization from the onset to the end of fatiguing contractions is even less. Tissue lactic acid concentration paralleled the glycogen depletion pattern. The concentration on tissue lactic acid while being highest at the point of fatigue for contractions between 30 and 50 percent MVC were substantially less than at the point of fatigue for contractions at 20 and 80 percent MVC, respectively. The lactic acid concentration at any tension was still substantially less than those reported to be found at the end of fatiguing dynamic exercise. The authors concluded, therefore, that muscle metabolism may not in itself have been a limiting factor in the fatigue process, except, perhaps, at the middle tensions, or it was possible that the metabolite that was associated with muscle fatigue may be some metabolite that they did not measure in the study. Similar findings were also reported by Edwards and his colleagues (1972) for skeletal muscle in the rat. Edwards et al. (1972) studied the concentration of several Krebs and glycolytic intermediates and ATP utilization, ATP concentration, PC concentration, and glycogen utilization in anoxic rat muscle during fatiguing isometric contractions. They also found the concentration of ATP at the point of fatigue to be higher than that which is found during dynamic exercise (Edwards et al. 1975). Further, they found glycogen utilization to be quite low during isometric contractions; however, they found a reduction in ATP turnover in fatigued muscle. This was also found by Bolstad and Ersland

(1978). In our own work, we found the tissue ATP, PC, lactic acid, and glycogen concentrations in the soleus (a slow-twitch muscle) and medial gastrocnemius (a fast-twitch muscle) to be fatigued during isometric contractions at tensions between 10–100 percent of the muscle's maximum strength (Petrofsky et al. 1979, 1980; Sawka et al. 1980). As reported by Edwards and Karlsson and their colleagues, we found that glycogen depletion was quite low during fatiguing isometric contractions at *any* tension we examined. During isometric contractions at any tension, the fast-twitch muscle (medial gastrocnemius) relied heavily on glycogen as a substrate during the contractions. This muscle

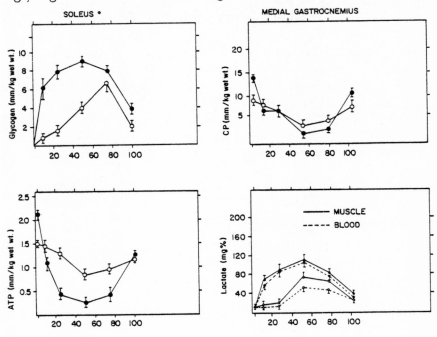

TENSION (% OF INITIAL STRENGTH)

Figure 5-1.   Muscle glycogen utilization, APT, PC, and lactate concentrations in six soleus and six medial gastrocnemius muscles ± SD at rest and at the end of fatiguing contractions. From Petrofsky, et al., Blood Flow and Metabolic Products During Fatiguing Isometric Contractions in Fast and Slow Skeletal Muscles in the Cat, *J Appl Physiol,* 50:493–502, 1981. Courtesy of The American Physiological Society.

showed the largest increase in lactic acid concentration and the greatest depletion in both glycogen and ATP at the point of fatigue following isometric contractions (*See* Figure 5-1). In contrast, for isometric contractions at low tensions (10–50% of the muscle strength), the soleus muscle appeared to use glucose and fatty acids as a substrate. Lactic acid production during these contractions was quite low, as was glycogen depletion. As tension was progressively increased during the fatiguing contractions, however, the soleus muscle began to depend heavily on aerobic pathways to produce energy. This was associated with an increase in glycogen utilization and in ATP degradation at the point of muscle fatigue (Sawka et al. 1980; Petrofsky et al. 1980). ATP turnover is much greater in fast- than slow-twitch muscle during fatiguing isometric contractions (Bolstad and Ersland 1978; Sawka et al. 1980). One curious finding was that in rat muscle depleted of phosphocreatine by β-guanidinoproprionate acid (Fitch et al. 1974), although there is a reduction in the maximum velocity of shortening of the slow-twitch muscles (Petrofsky and Fitch 1980), isometric (Fitch et al 1974; Petrofsky and Fitch 1980) endurance was not altered in fast-twitch muscle and tripled in slow-twitch muscle pointing to the independence of the fatigue process on tissue energy stores.

MECHANICAL PROPERTIES OF FATIGUED MUSCLE

Associated with fatigue from sustained submaximal isometric contractions is a change in the mechanical properties of the muscle. Twitch tension decreases, and the rate of rise and fall of tension during an isometric twitch increases at the end of a fatiguing isometric contraction (Petrofsky et al. 1979; Petrofsky and Fitch 1980.) Further, previously active muscle exhibits post-tetanic potentiation partially due to an increased release of Ach at the neuromuscular junction (Liley and North 1953). Finally, Edwards et al. (1972) and Petrofsky et al. (1980) have reported a reduction in ATPase activity associated with fatiguing isometric contractions. In experiments in cat skeletal muscle, Petrofsky et al. (1980) showed a reduction in Vmax at the point of isometric fatigue (*see* Figure 5-2). Since Vmax has been correlated to the ATPase of actin and myosin, the implication is that there is a re-

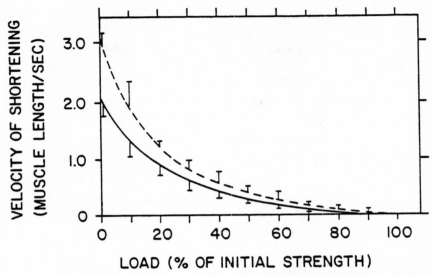

Figure 5-2.   Relationship of velocity of shortening to load. Means ± SD are shown for six control soleus (dashed line) and six phosphocreatine-depleted soleus muscles (solid line). From Petrofsky and Fitch, Contractile Characteristics of Skeletal Muscle Depleted of Phosphocreatinine, *Eur J Physiol*, *384*:123–129, 1980. Courtesy of Springer-Verlag New York, Inc.

duction in actomyosin ATPase at the point of fatigue.

Muscle metabolism during isometric exercise appears to depend largely on the temperature of the exercising muscles. In man, it has been shown that the temperature of the exercising muscle can vary widely. For example, for the brachioradialus muscle, the resting, deep muscle temperature of an individual in a thermally neutral environment, with his arms bared to the shoulder, is about 32° C. (Clarke, Hellon, and Lind 1958; Petrofsky and Lind 1975B). Increasing or decreasing the environmental temperature will alter muscle temperature dramatically. When muscle contracts isometrically at temperatures between 22°–25° C, the degradation in tissue glycogen and ATP utilization at the point of isometric fatigue is substantially less than that which occurs at the warmer muscle temperatures (Petrofsky et al. 1980; Edwards et al. 1972). However, although some neuromuscular block has been shown to be associated with the cold (Cullingham, Lind, and Morton 1965), by and large, over the muscle temperature range of 22°–38° C, fatigue appears to be largely in the contractile components in the muscle (Petrofsky and Lind 1980). Although Cullingham, Lind, and Morton did find significant failure of the neuromuscular junctions in the cold, the frequency of stimulation used in their studies was far above the physiological range.

CENTRAL VS. PERIPHERAL FATIGUE

Certainly, in many of the muscle metabolism studies cited here, it would appear that energy depletion was not the limiting factor resulting in fatigue from isometric exercise. However, since there is a reduction in actomyosin ATPase associated with isometric fatigue, the buildup of some metabolite limiting the viability of actomyosin cross bridges cannot be ruled out.

Certainly, the concept of fatigue originating in the central nervous system has been well established (Reid 1928; Simonson 1972). Isometric contractions are typically quite painful to sustain to fatigue. Therefore, there is a great deal of motivation involved in sustaining an isometric contraction. Rodbard and Pragay (1968) proposed that isometric fatigue was pain limited, and a fatigue index could be developed in terms of five levels of pain associated with exerting isometric contractions. Further, Ikai and Steinhaus (1972) and several other investigators have shown that in some subjects simply shouting at the subject can increase isometric strength and endurance. However, as cited in Chapter 1 on *Isometric Training,* in well-motivated subjects, even hypnosis could not increase isometric strength and endurance, for example Barber 1966. Therefore, in well-motivated subjects, cortical influences on fatigue can probably be ruled out. However, it is possible that some fatigue may develop within the spinal cord or in the alphamotor neurons as proposed by Krnjevic and Miledi (1959). Krnjevic and Miledi found that in the rat diaphragm there was failure to propagate action potentials on the alpha motorneurons at the point where the nerve branches into the muscle. Studies of the electrical activity of muscle during voluntary isometric contractions have provided evidence to support this hypothesis. Stephens and Taylor (1972) found that during a sustained maximal voluntary effort there was a parallel fall in the average amplitude of the electromyogram (EMG) and force for the first 3–5 minutes that the contraction was sustained. After this point in time the electrical activity for the muscle plateaued, while tension continually fell. They felt that in the initial 3–5 minutes of a sustained maximal effort, the parallel fall in both the electrical activity and tension showed either fatigue in the central nervous system (e.g. spinal cord) at the neuromuscular junction or the failure of the sarcolemma to propagate action potentials. Further evidence of this nature is also found during sustained submaximal isometric contractions. During submaximal isometric contractions, the EMG amplitude increases continuously throughout the duration of the contractions (*See* Chapter 3). However, at the point of isometric fatigue, the amplitude of the surface electromyogram is linearly related to the tension exerted during the contractions. For example, when subjects sustain a tension of 70 percent MVC to fatigue, the electromyogram at the point of fatigue is equal in amplitude to that during an MVC in fresh muscle. In contrast, for contractions sustained at 25 percent MVC at the point of fatigue, the amplitude of the surface electromyogram is only equal to about half of that of an MVC in the fresh muscle (Lind and Petrofsky 1979). The simplest conclusion that can be drawn from these data is that the contractions associated with low tension isometric contractions (e.g. 25% MVC) are associated with some sort of electrical failure in the muscle or in the central nervous system (*See* Figure 5-3). However, Ochs et al. (1977), Mortimer, Magnusson, and Petersen (1970), and Petrofsky et al. (1978, 1980) have all examined the amplitude of muscle action potentials during sustained submaximal isometric contractions. During sustained submaximal isometric contractions the amplitude of the motor unit action potentials is not significantly altered throughout the duration of the contractions. Further, Bigland-Ritchie and her colleagues (1978, 1979, 1980) also found that the amplitude of the action potentials recorded from skeletal muscle fibers during a sustained maximal effort was not substantially reduced from control values. However, Petrofsky (1981) and Bigland-Ritchie and Lippold (1980) and Bigland-Richie et al.

(1980) found the frequency of discharge at the point of isometric fatigue for contractions sustained at submaximal tensions and during a sustained maximal effort, respectively, was lower than that recorded in unfatigued muscle during an MVC. This then would seem to imply that fatigue may occur either within the central nervous system or in a failure to propagate action potentials across the motor nerve or muscle fiber when muscle fatigues at low submaximal isometric tensions or during a sustained maximal effort. However, Petrofsky (1980) and Bigland-Ritchie and Lippold (1980) both found that muscles were able to respond quite adequately to electrical stimulation at normal physiological frequencies when fatigued under the circumstances, although muscle does become refractory to high-frequency electrical stimulation when fatigued isometrically (Brown and Burns 1949; Jones et al. 1979; Petrofsky, 1980; Bigland-Ritchie and Lippold 1980; Bigland-Ritchie et al. 1978, 1980). The inescapable conclusion then is that there is some fatigue within the central nervous system under these experimental circumstances. For example, when fatiguing submaximal isometric contractions are sustained at tensions between 25 and 55 percent MVC, and the motor unit discharge frequencies are measured throughout the duration of the contractions, the relationship between the final motor unit discharge frequency and tension is shown in Figure 5-4. For submaximal isometric contractions there is a linear relationship between the tension exerted during the contractions and the final motor unit discharge frequency. It has long been established in muscle physiology (Guyton, 1980) that tension developed by skeletal muscle is sensitive to the frequency of stimulation. For example, when a muscle, such as the medial gastrocnemius muscle in the cat, is stimulated by a single pair of electrodes at various frequencies between 2 Hz and 200 Hz, and the tension developed by the muscle is measured, a typical frequency relationship is shown (*See* Figure 5-5). The general shape of this curve is S-shaped. As the stimulation frequency is increased between 2 Hz and 100 Hz there is a rapid rise in the tension developed by the muscle. Varying the frequency of motor unit discharge is one mechanism by which the body can adjust the tension developed by the muscle (Bigland and Lippold 1954B; Milner-Brown and Stein 1975). It can be proposed then that lower discharge frequencies in the fatigued muscle will result in less tension developed by the muscle. This will then support the observations by Lind and Petrofsky (1979) and by Stephens and Taylor (1972) in that the lower maximum tension developed by the skeletal muscle at the point of fatigue during light isometric contractions and during sustained maximal efforts, respectively, could be accounted for in terms of central muscle fatigue. However, Brown and Burns (1949), Petrofsky (1980), Petrofsky and Fitch (1979) and Edwards et al. (1975) have all shown that fatigued skeletal muscle can tetanize at lower discharge frequencies than is found for fresh muscle. Therefore, if the skeletal muscle is fatigued isometrically, as shown for a cat medial gastrocnemius muscle in Figure 5-6, the frequency tension relationship shifts to the left. As can be seen in this figure, muscles are able to tetanize at substantially lower frequencies after being fatigued isometrically.

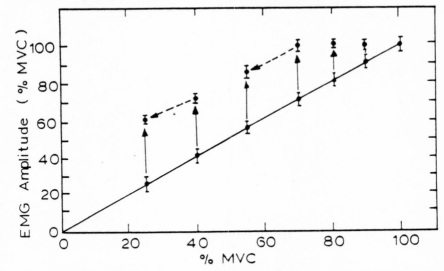

Figure 5-3.   The amplitude of the surface EMG at the onset (solid line) and throughout the duration of fatiguing isometric contractions at submaximal tensions. From Lind and Petrofsky, Amplitude of the Electromyogram During Fatiguing Isometric Contractions, *Muscle and Nerve*, 2:257–324, 1979. Courtesy of John Wiley & Sons, Inc.

Therefore, although lower discharge frequencies arise from the alpha motor neuron pool, these discharge frequencies may be totally unrelated to the fatigue developed by the skeletal muscle. Further, the small changes in the amplitude and duration of ac-

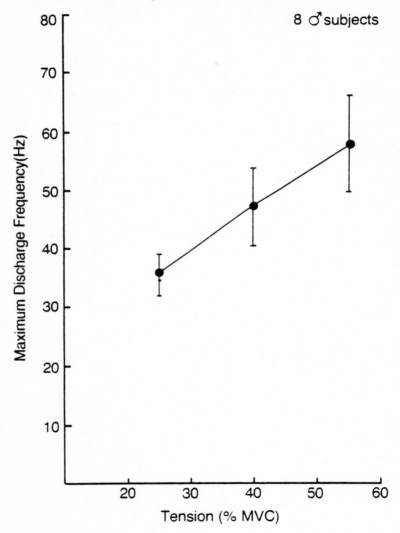

Figure 5-4.   The average discharge frequency of motor units in the adductor pollicis muscle of four male subjects at the end of fatiguing isometric contractions at 25, 40, and 55 percent MVC.

tion potentials associated with fatiguing isometric contractions have been shown to have little effect on the contractile tension developed by the skeletal muscle, as well (Fink and Luttgau 1976). The mechanism of the reduction in discharge frequency associated with fatiguing isometric exercise may simply be related to afferent input from sensory receptors on the alpha motor neuron pool. Grimby and Hannerz (1976) and Hannerz and Grimby (1979) have shown that proprioceptive activity can alter the discharge frequency of motor neurons in the alpha motor neuron pool. Therefore, it is not surprising that during sustained isometric contractions there may be some effect of muscle tension on the frequency of discharge of the alpha motor neuron pool. However, for arguments cited previously, this lower discharge frequency has no apparent effect on the contractile tension developed by skeletal muscle (Petrofsky 1980; Merton 1954).

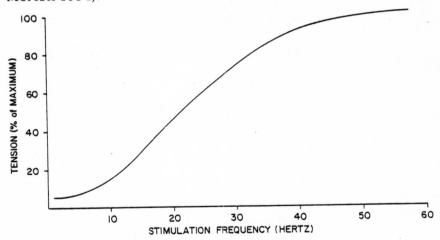

Figure 5-5.   A typical frequency-tension relationship for skeletal muscle.

CONCLUSIONS

From the data included in this chapter it would appear that fatigue is a very complex process in skeletal muscle during isometric contractions. Although some differences occur in the motor unit discharge properties associated with fatiguing

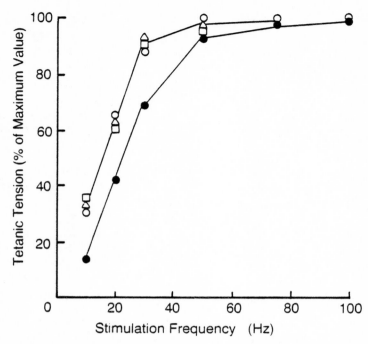

Figure 5-6.   The frequency tension in fresh (●) and fatigued muscle. From Petrofsky et al., Mechanical and Electrical Correlates of Isometric Muscle Fatigue in Skeletal Muscle in the Cat, *Eur J Physiol*, *387*:33–38, 1980. Courtesy of Springer-Verlag New York, Inc.

isometric contractions at various tensions, the inescapable conclusion of this work is that *muscle fatigue probably resides in the skeletal muscle.* However, energy depletion is far from complete during fatiguing isometric contractions, particularly at low and high tensions. The reduction in actomyosin ATPase and ATP turnover associated with fatiguing exercise would seem to imply some molecular event in the contractile mechanism associated with muscle fatigue. Since the usual metabolites associated with isometric exercise (e.g. ATP, PC, glycogen, lactic acid) cannot be held responsible for the fatigue process, it is possible that some as yet unidentified metabolite is associated with muscle fatigue during isometric contractions. Further work is necessary in this area to establish which metabolite is involved.

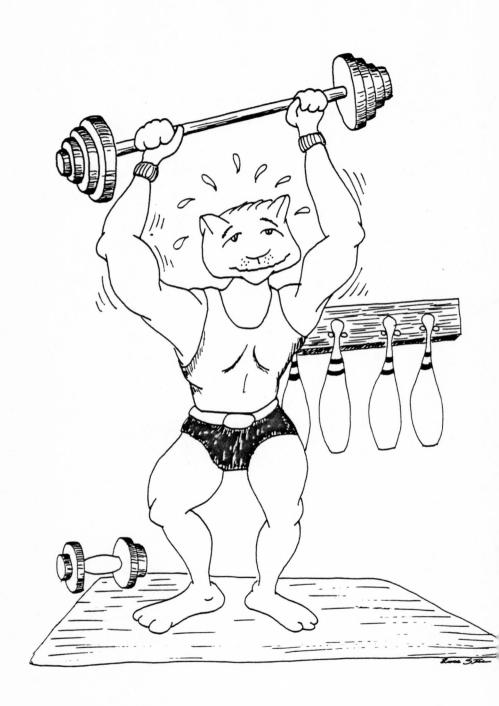

CHAPTER 6

THE INTERRELATIONSHIPS BETWEEN STATIC AND DYNAMIC EXERCISE

$\mathbf{A}$lthough isometric exercise is easy to perform in a laboratory situation, it is much less common to find pure isometric exercise in an industrial setting. Likewise, pure dynamic exercise is also rarely performed. Generally, most exercise is a mixture of static and dynamic exercise. For example, walking is a mixture of both static and dynamic exercise. While some muscles contract and relax isotonically, others must contract isometrically to fix the joints of the body so that upright posture can be maintained. Riding a bicycle is another form of a mixed static and dynamic exercise, since isometric contractions are exerted by the hands to hold the handles of the bicycle while the legs are exercising dynamically. In both of these brief examples, some muscle groups were exerting static contractions while others were exerting dynamic contractions.

But the situation in real life can be even far more complex. When people work at low rates against a heavy load, the exercise is neither pure static nor pure dynamic, but in fact contains elements of both. Dynamic exercise at a light load and high speed is said to have a low static component and be almost pure dynamic exercise, whereas slow contractions against a heavy load are said to have a high static component. It will be the purpose of this chapter to explore the fatigue characteristics of skeletal muscle and the associated cardiorespiratory reflexes during combined static and dynamic exercise and during dynamic exercise with a high static component.

COMBINED STATIC AND DYNAMIC EXERCISE

As described in previous chapters, isometric exercise, while

113

being associated with short endurance, results in a potent systolic and diastolic blood pressure response and a modest increase in heart rate throughout the duration of fatiguing contractions. In contrast, during dynamic exercise (when the exercise is sustained at high levels) there is a large increase in heart rate but generally only a small change in mean blood pressure throughout the duration of the exercise. When static and dynamic exercise are performed together, the individual cardiovascular responses of the two types of exercise are additive. The interrelationships between simultaneous static and dynamic exercise were first explored by Wiley and Lind (1971). In these studies, Wiley and Lind investigated isometric endurance and the ventilatory responses to isometric handgrip contractions done simultaneously with bicycling on the Monarch bicycle® ergometer. They found that when an isometric handgrip contraction was performed during bicycling the endurance was longer than

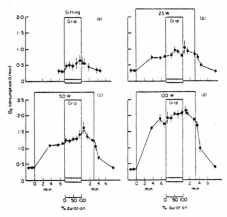

Figure 6-1.   Oxygen consumption (mean values ± SEM, l/min) of six subjects in four conditions: (1) fatiguing handgrip contraction (grip) while sitting on the bicycle ergometer (a); (2) grip superimposed during a period of rhythmic exercise on the bicycle ergometer at 25 W (b), 50 W(c), and 100 W(d). Time during periods of cycling alone is expressed in minutes. Time during grip periods is expressed as percent of the duration to fatigue, so normalizing duration of grip, which ranged from 138 to 181 seconds. From Wiley and Lind, Respiratory Responses to Sustained Static Muscular Contractions in Humans, *Clin Sci, 40*:221–234, 1971. Courtesy of Biochemical Society.

when the isometric contraction was performed in the absence of bicycling. The mechanism of this response was attributed to the increased blood pressure during the dynamic exercise. During an isometric contraction, the increased intramuscular pressure either fully or partially occludes the blood flow to the handgrip muscles. The precise tension at which occlusion occurs appears to vary in different muscles in the body. Barcroft and Millen (1939) studied the calf muscles and concluded that the limiting tension was about 20 – 30 percent MVC. They felt that the blood flow was occluded due to the mechanical nipping of the arteries in the facial sheath surrounding the muscle. In contrast, Lind et al. (1964) found that blood flow was occluded for the forearm muscles only at tensions exceeding 70 percent MVC. Here it was felt that occlusion occurred due to constriction of the arterials resulting from high intramuscular pressure during the contractions (Grey et al. 1967). Since Wiley and Lind (1971) had their

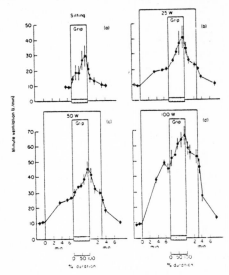

Figure 6-2.   Minute ventilation (mean values ± SEM, l/min) for six subjects. Time during periods of cycling alone is expressed in minutes. Time during grip periods is expressed as percent of the duration to fatigue, as described for Figure 6-1. From Wiley and Lind, Respiratory Responses to Sustained Static Muscular Contractions in Humans, *Clin Sci, 40*:221–234, 1971. Courtesy of Biochemical Society.

subjects perform contractions at 40 percent MVC, although intramuscular pressure is high, blood still perfuses the muscle.
Therefore, an increased arterial pressure due to the dynamic
exercise would increase perfusion of the muscle and result in an
increase in isometric endurance.

During isometric contractions, the increase in oxygen consumption above rest is small (Wiley and Lind 1971). This also
holds true for isometric handgrip contractions conducted during dynamic exercise, as shown in Figure 6-1. In contrast, the increase in minute ventilation (*See* Figures 6-2 and 6-3) is generally
found to be disproportionately large to the increase in oxygen

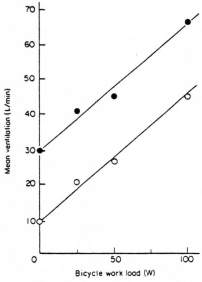

Figure 6-3.   Mean minute ventilation responses to cycling with (●), and without (○), static handgrip. Work loads are shown along the abscissa
in watts and minute ventilation along the ordinate in l/min. Zero
work load represents experiments with subjects seated on the
bicycle ergometer, not cycling. ○ values are taken from Figure 6-2
and represent the last measurement before commencing the
handgrip effort; ● values represent the last measurement in the
"grip" period; lines were drawn by eye. From Wiley and Lind,
Respiratory Responses to Sustained Static Muscular Contractions
in Humans, *Clin Sci, 40*:221–234, 1971. Courtesy of Biochemical
Society.

consumption during isometric handgrip alone or performed during cycling. As might be expected, then, there is a marked hyperventilation during static exercise alone or combined static and dynamic exercise (Figure 6-4) as assessed by the ventilatory equivalent.

When the isometric handgrip contractions are performed during dynamic exercise, Kilbrom (1976, 1978) found that the heart rate response to the combined exercise was almost equal to the summation of the individual heart rate responses recorded when the two individual forms of exercise were done alone (Figure 6-5). This was also true of the blood pressure response, since the blood pressure response during the isometric exercise was simply superimposed on that of dynamic exercise (Figure 6-6).

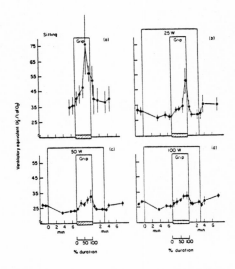

Figure 6-4. Ventilatory equivalent (mean values ± sem) for six subjects. Time during periods of cycling alone is expressed in minutes. Time during grip periods is expressed as percent of the duration to fatigue, as described for Figure 6-1.From Wiley and Lind, Respiratory Responses to Sustained Static Muscular Contractions in Humans, *Clin Sci, 40*:221–234, 1971. Courtesy of Biochemical Society.

STATIC COMPONENT OF DYNAMIC EXERCISE

The static component of dynamic exercise has been difficult to quantify. The efficiency of dynamic exercise such as bicycling is generally about 30 percent (Petrofsky and Lind 1978; Petrofsky et al. 1975). However, if dynamic work is performed slowly and under a heavy load, the efficiency drops dramatically (Benedict and Cathcart 1913; Dickinson 1929, Petrofsky 1975, et al.; Petrofsky and Lind 1978). For example, during slow lifting of lead boxes from the floor to tabletop level, the efficiency was always less than 10 percent in both male and female subjects. (Petrofsky

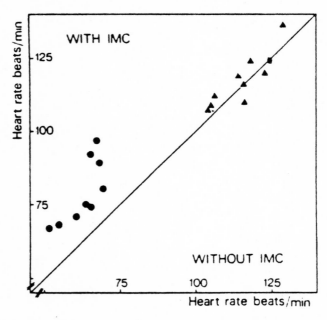

Figure 6-5.   Heart rate with and without sustained isometric contraction (IMC). On the abscissa, individual values obtained at supine rest (●) or during dynamic leg exercise (▲) are given. The ordinate gives results obtained in the same subjects during IMC performed separately (●) or in combination with dynamic leg exercise (▲). Measurements were made after four minutes of activity. From Kilbrom, Circulatory and Ventilatory Effects of Combined Static and Dynamic Activities, *Scand J Rehab Med*, 10:99–104, 1978. Courtesy of National Board of Occupational Safety and Health.

and Lind 1978); Williams, Petrofsky, and Lind 1981; Lind, Williams, and Petrofsky 1981). This reduction in mechanical efficiency was first used by Atzler (1925) to quantify fatigue. Assuming that muscle had an efficiency of 30 percent during pure dynamic exercise, Atzler and his colleagues calculated the partial mechanical efficiency (N_5) as the theoretical efficiency of doing a task (30%) minus the energy cost for movement without a load (Leerbewegung). A comparison of the partial mechanical efficiency (N_5) during various types of work with varying static components showed generally good agreement between N_5 and the subjective feelings of the subjects for the static component. Although mechanical efficiency increases in the first few minutes of work (Simonson and Hebestreit 1930; Simonson 1936; Müller

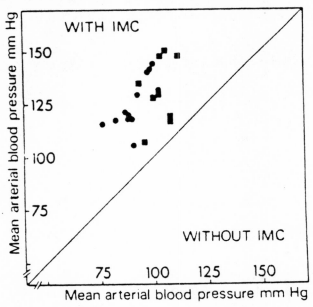

Figure 6-6. Effect on mean intra-arterial blood pressure of sustained IMC performed separately or in combination with dynamic exercise. Each symbol represents one subject. ● = Comparison between supine rest and isolated IMC. ■ = Comparison between dynamic leg exercise and combined dynamic and isometric exercise. From Kilbrom, Circulatory and Ventilatory Effects of Combined Static and Dynamic Activities, *Scand J Rehab Med, 10*:99–104, 1978. Courtesy of National Board of Occupational Safety and Health.

and Hettinger 1953), there was no consistent effect of static component on this "warm up" phenomenon. In most experiments, RQ appears to increase during dynamic work (Dusser de Barenne and Van Burger 1928). In addition, when work has a high static component, there is generally a hyperventilation (Wiley and Lind 1971), but no consistent relationships between O_2 debt or O_2 deficit has been found associated with the static

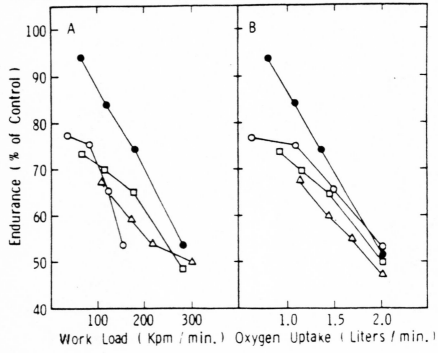

Figure 6-7. Isometric endurance at tension of 40 percent MVC following 1-hour bouts of lifting. Data are normalized on ordinate to control endurance times (as average of three separate contractions for each subject) on days when they were not involved on lifting experiments. Illustrated are isometric endurances of hand-grip muscles after lifting 6.82 (○), 22.73 (□), and 36.36 (△) kilogram boxes for one-hour as well as endurance for isometric exercise of arm and back muscles following one-hour bouts of lifting the 22.73 kilogram boxes (●). From Petrofsky and Lind, Metabolic, Cardiovascular and Respiratory Factors in the Development of Fatigue in Lifting Tasks, *J Appl Physiol, 45*:270–274, 1978. Courtesy of The American Physiological Society.

component of dynamic exercise. However, Simonson (1927) did show a faster recovery of oxidative capacity following work with a high static component. Petrofsky et al. (1975) developed a technique to quantify the static component of dynamic exercise. Briefly, the technique involved having subjects exert a fatiguing isometric contraction following a bout of dynamic exercise. When isometric contractions of the quadriceps muscle followed dynamic exercise, whose work load was set to require 25, 50 and 70 percent of the $\dot{V}O_2$ max at a cycling speed of 90 RPM, it was found for work loads below 50 percent of the $\dot{V}O_2$ max, dynamic exercise had little effect on static endurance. However, as the dynamic load was increased, static endurance was progressively reduced. Obviously, a dynamic work load at a speed of 90 RPM would have been almost pure dynamic exercise and have a very low static component. In contrast, intuitively, work loads requiring the same percent of the $\dot{V}O_2$ max but where the cycling speed was 30 RPM would involve cycling against very heavy static loads. When the static endurance of contractions performed after cycling at 90 RPM was compared to those performed after cycling at 30 RPM at similar dynamic work levels, the increased static load resulted in a substantial fall in isometric endurance (Petrofsky et al. 1975). In this manner, then, the static component of dynamic exercise can be quantified. Using this technique, the static component during lifting weights has also been quantified for the lower back and arm muscles; similar observations were found. For example, when lifting boxes (Petrofsky and Lind 1978) from floor to table height it has been shown that, even at the same dynamic work load, lifting involving heavy weights at slow rates resulted in substantially less isometric endurance than lifting weights at high rates and low rates for both the forearms and lower back muscles as shown in this figure (*See* Figure 6-7).

But dynamic exercise can alter the recovery from static exercise as well. Often, in the industrial or military setting, periods of intense static exercise are alternated with periods of light to moderate dynamic exercise. One typical example is seen in air-

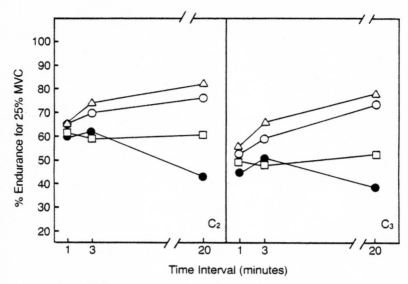

Figure 6-8.　Isometric endurance for the third of a series of isometric contractions normalized in terms of the first isometric contraction. During the intercontraction interval of 1, 3, or 20 minutes the subjects rested ($\triangle$) or bicycled at 0 kp ($\triangle$) or a load that required 50 ($\square$) or 75 percent ($\bullet$) VO_2 max.

craft pilots during flight maneuvers under varying G loads where periods of light dynamic work with heavy static contractions are alternated. The effect of dynamic work on the recovery from fatiguing isometric contractions has been recently explored by Fiori, (1980). Dynamic exercise at levels of less than 50 percent of the VO_2 max has little effect on the recovery following isometric exercise (Figure 8) for periods up to twenty minutes (*See* Figure 6-8). In contrast, dynamic exercise reduces the recovery following fatiguing isometric exercise if the level of the work exceeds 50 percent of the $\dot{V}O_2$ max.

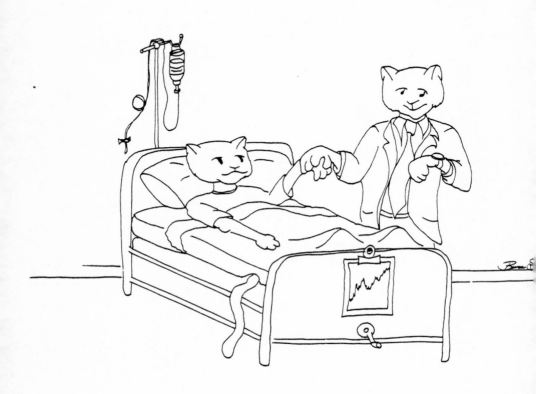

CHAPTER 7

CLINICAL IMPLICATIONS OF
ISOMETRIC EXERCISE

ISOMETRIC EXERCISE AND THE HEART

For the normal heart isometric exercise poses a unique stress. Unlike dynamic exercise, where cardiac output increases dramatically with typically no change in mean blood pressure, during isometric exercise cardiac output increases only slightly, but mean blood pressure increases dramatically (Lind et al. 1964). This results in a sharp increase in the afterload on the heart. For the normal myocardium this appears to create no problem. However, in the diseased myocardium, blood pressure typically increases the same as is found in the normal individual. However, due to a reduced coronary blood flow reserve, coronary blood flow does not increase in proportion to the load imposed on the heart (Miyazowa et al. 1977). The increased afterload associated with isometric exercise has been shown to precipitate many of the symptoms of congestive heart failure in many individuals with a diseased myocardium. These symptoms include, for example, a sharp increase in left ventricular end-diastolic blood pressure LVEDP during isometric contractions (Miyazowa et al. 1980). In the normal patient at the end of a fatiguing isometric contraction, the left ventricular end-diastolic blood pressure is usually about 5 mm Hg. In contrast, in a diseased myocardium, left ventricular end-diastolic blood pressure has been shown to rise between 25 and 50 mm Hg. Further, although left ventricular end-diastolic volume increases during isometric exercise in both normals and patients with heart disease, the velocity of shortening of the myocardial fibers increases during isometric exercise in normals but stays constant in patients with heart disease. Finally, stroke work, while increasing in normals, does not increase appreciably during isometric exercise in coronary patients (Mitchell 1974; Krayenbuehl et al. 1972). The implication is that in patients with coronary disease, the Frank-Starling mechanism must be used to increase the blood pressure (Miyazowa et al. 1980; Krayenbuehl 1973; Mullins et al. · 1970; Helfant et al. 1971; Kivowitz et al. 1971). If the myocardial disease involves the heart valves, isometric exercise may be accompanied by a pronounced increase in heart sounds and murmurs (Hume et al. 1978). In patients with arterioschlerotic heart disease, for example, isometric exercise increases the third and fourth heart sounds (Matthews et al. 1970). In patients with aortic stenosis, isometric exercise has been helpful in altering the murmurs to distinguish this disease from subaortic obstruction (Mosseler et al. 1971).

For this reason, because of the unique stress placed on the heart by isometric exercise, many hospitals have incorporated an isometric stress test either in combination with or separate from a treadmill stress test for the diagnosis of myocardial abnormalities (Helfant et al. 1971; Kivowitz et al. 1971; Krayenbuehl et al. 1972; Fisher et al. 1973; Grossman et al. 1973; Quinones et al. 1974; Houston et al. 1970; Siegal et al. 1972). Although some individuals may show abnormalities in either the ECG or heart sounds during both treadmill and isometric stress testing, typically, individuals will show abnormalities in either one or the other type of test, but rarely both. Systolic time intervals during isometric exercise are not altered by coronary disease (Houston et al. 1970; Siegal et al. 1972.)

Because of the simplicity in instrumentation involved in this type of study, and the lack of movement involved on the part of the patient, this type of exercise is particularly easy to accomplish on the cardiac catheterization table. If the heart rate is held constant by using a pacemaker, stroke work index increases markedly while LVEDP changes little. In contrast, in the patient with heart disease, stroke work usually stays constant during pacing while LVEDP increases (Amande et al. 1972). It would appear, then, that isometric stress testing might be a useful clinical tool for noninvasive studies of cardiovascular function, since it offers an easy means of increasing the load on the heart. However, in patients with angina, dynamic exercise precipitates pain in some patients in which static exercise may not (Jackson 1970; Siegal et al. 1972). In contrast, in other studies (Baccelli et al. 1978) the reverse is true, and the isometric handgrip precipitates ischemic changes in the ECG (Nyberg et al. 1979). In patients recovering from myocardial infarctions, isometric exercise has been shown to be useful in unmasking impairment of ventricular function that was not evident in the resting subject (Baccelli et al. 1978). In summary, since the stress of isometric exercise on the heart is so very different from dynamic exercise, a good stress test would probably include both tests.

Isometric stress testing has proven to be particularly useful in predicting the survivability of patients following heart transplant. During isometric exercise in the denervated heart (heart transplant), the systolic and diastolic blood pressure increase to the same level as in the normally innervated heart (Savin et al. 1980). Patients who survive dynamic stress tests, but fail isometric stress tests prior to heart transplant, have been shown to have a much higher mortality rate than occurs for patients who either pass or fail the dynamic stress test but pass the isometric stress test. In both groups of patients, following heart transplant, the patients were able to pass the isometric stress test.

One of the reasons that isometric exercise may be so dangerous for the unstable myocardium may lie in the mechanism used by the body to increase heart rate during this form of exertion. Heart rate during isometric exercise is increased entirely due to withdrawal of vagal tone. Corr (1975) and Corr and Gillis (1974) have shown that following a myocardial infarction the heart becomes electrically unstable. In human and animal experiments, they have found that the survival rate was lowest when vagal traffic was also low. By using parasympathetic memonic agents to increase vagal tone, survival could be dramatically increased. In contrast, reducing vagal tone by parasympathectomy of the heart or blocking parasympathetic activity of the heart with pharmaceutical agents generally resulted in electrical instability and myocardial fibrillation. It is possible that the reduction in vagal traffic associated with isometric exercise may cause electrical instability in the diseased myocardium and may result in the poor tolerance seen for isometric exercise after an acute myocardial infarction in these individuals (Perez et al. 1980).

One complicating problem associated with static work is an enhanced platelet aggregation following isometric exercise in patients with ischemic coronary disease. This may predispose blood clot formation on the heart (Sano et al. 1977, 1980). This effect can be blocked by dipyridamole.

Finally, the consequence of isometric exercise on a patient with an aneurysm must not be overlooked. Because of the increase in blood pressure associated with isometric exercise, this form of exercise may precipitate the destruction of an aneurysm on a blood vessel. This might be particularly the case in people who are hypertensive.

HYPERTENSION AND ISOMETRIC EXERCISE

In studies of normal individuals, it has been shown that the blood pressure at the end of a fatiguing isometric contraction is highly correlated to the blood pressure at the onset of the contraction. For example, if in any one day a subject enters a laboratory with the resting blood pressure elevated 10 mm Hg above normal, the blood presure at the end of the isometric contraction will also be elevated by 10 mm Hg above normal. The same situation applies to the hypertensive patient. For the hypertensive patient, due to a wide variety of etiologies including hyperthyroidism, it has been shown that the blood pressure at the end of the isometric contraction will increase by 50 percent over the resting pressure, irrespective of the resting pressure at the onset of the contraction. Blood pressure as high as 350/200 mm Hg have been reported at the end of isometric contractions in hypertensive patients (Hoel et al. 1970; Ewing et al. 1973; Reubon et al. 1979; Fixler et al. 1979; Chrysant 1978; Nudel et al. 1980).

Ewing (1973) reported that ventricular function of hypertensive patients can be divided into two groups. In some patients there is an increase in peripheral resistance and little increase in cardiac output. While in others, peripheral resistance increases little while cardiac output increases. While the heart rate response to isometric exercise is lowered by a β blocking agent (Propranolol®), neither alpha (Prazosin®) nor β blocking agents in clinical doses were able to lower the pressor response during isometric exercise in hypertensive patients (essential) (Reubon et al. 1979; McAllister 1979), although blocking agents did lower the pressor response in normal subjects. Large doses of blocking agents given intravenously were able to abolish the response. This situation is exaggerated even further in the elderly, who have a higher rate of rise of blood pressure and a higher absolute increase in blood pressure during isometric contractions, due to the presence of atherosclerosis (Petrofsky and Lind 1975; Ordwam and Wekstein 1979).

Given this, it is surprising that isometric exercise has been recommended as treatment for hypertension (Kiveloff and Huber 1971). In the adolescent with hypertension, abnormalities in ECG are not seen during dynamic or static exercise (Fixler et al. 1979; Stentler et al. 1979; Nudel et al. 1980). However, it is apparent that this form of exercise would be dangerous for the elderly hypertensive patient. In hypertensive patients, one complicating factor is the effect of isometric handgrip on the kidneys. In these patients, isometric handgrip is associated with a retention of Na^+ and K^+ for hours after isometric exercise (Parfrey et al. 1979), which can further aggravate the problem.

BIBLIOGRAPHY

Alam, M., and Smirk, F.H. Observations in man upon a blood pressure raising reflex arising from the voluntary muscles. *J Physiol, 89*:372–383, 1937.

—————— Observations in man on a pulse-accelerating reflex from the voluntary muscles of the legs. *J Physiol, 92*:167–177, 1938.

—————— Unilateral loss of a blood pressure raising, pulse accelerating, reflex from voluntary muscle due to a lesion of the spinal cord. *Clin Sci, 3*:247–252, 1938.

Amende, I., Krayenbuehl, H.P., Rutishauser, W., and Wirz, P. Left ventricular dynamics during handgrip. *Br Heart J, 34*:688–695, 1972.

Ariano, M.A., Armstrong, R.B., and Edgerton, V.R. Hindlimb muscle fiber populations of five mammals, *J of Histochem and Cytochem, 21*(1):51–55, 1973.

Asmussen, E., and Hansen, E. Studies on isometric exercise. *Scand Arch Physiol, 78*:283–303, 1938.

—————— Studies on static work. *Scand Arch Physiol, 77*:6–17, 1937.

Astrand, P.O., and Rodahl, K. *Textbook of Work Physiology.* New York: McGraw-Hill, 1970.

Atzler, E., Herbst, R., Lehmann, G., and Muller, E. Arbeitsphysiologische Studien. *Pfluegers Arch, 208*:184–191, 1925.

Baccelli, G., Valentini, R., Cellina, G.G., Mancia, G., Ludbrook, J., and Zanchetti, A. Haemodynamic effects of isometric handgrip exercise in patients convalescent from myocardial infarction. *Clin Exp Pharmacol Physiol, 5*:607–615, 1978.

Barany, M., and Close, R. The transformation of myosin in cross-innervated rat muscles. *J Physiol, 213*:455–474, 1971.

Barber, T.X. The effects of hypnosis and motivated suggestions on strength and endurance: a critical review of research studies. *Brit J Soc Clin Physiol, 5*:42–56, 1966.

Barcroft, H. An inquiry into the nature of the mediator of the vasodilitation of skeletal muscle in exercise and during circulatory arrest. *J Physiol, 222*:99P, 1972.

Barcroft, H. and Edholm, O. The effect of temperature on blood flow and deep muscle temperature in the human forearm. *J Physiol, 102*:5–17, 1943.

—————— Temperature and blood flow in the human forearm. *J Physiol, 104*:366–376, 1946.

Barcroft, H., and Millen, J.E. Blood flow through muscle during sustained contractions. *J Physiol, 97*:17–31, 1939.

Barnard, R.J., Edgerton, V.R., and Peter, J.B. Effect of exercise on skeletal muscle. I. Biochemical and histochemical properties. *J Appl Physiol, 28*:762–766, 1970.

Barnard, R.J., and Peter, J.B. Effect of training and exhaustion on hexokinase activity of skeletal muscle. *J Appl Physiol, 27*:691–695, 1969.

Benedict, F., and Cathcart, E.P. *Muscular Work*, Publ. No. 187, Carnegie Institute of Washington, 1913.

Bergenwald, L., Eklund, B., and Freyschuss, U. Effect of acute blood volume variations in man on the circulatory response to isometric handgrip. *Scand J Clin Lab Invest, 37*:683–689, 1977.

Berger, R.A. Effects of knowledge of isometric strength during performance on recorded strength. *Res Q, 38*:507–519, 1967.

Bigland, B. and Lippold, O.C.J. The relation between force, velocity and integrated electrical activity in human muscles. *J Physiol, 123*:214–224, 1954.

———— Motor unit activity in the voluntary contraction of human muscle. *J Physiol, 125*:322–335, 1954.

Bigland-Ritchie, B., Jones, D.A., Hosking, G.P., and Edwards, R.H.T. Central and peripheral fatigue in sustained maximum voluntary contractions of human quadriceps muscle. *Clin Sci Mol Med., 54*:609–614, 1978.

Bigland-Ritchie, B., and Lippold, O.C.S. Changes in muscle activation during prolonged maximal voluntary contractions. *J Physiol*, 14, 1979.

Bigland-Ritchie, B. and Lippold, O.C.J. Neuromuscular block and motor firing frequencies in human muscular fatigue. *Proc Int Physiol Soc, 14*:326, 1980.

Bockman, E.L., Berne, R.M., and Rubio, R. Adenosine and active hyperemia in dog skeletal muscle. *Am J Physiol, 230*:1531–1537, 1976.

Bodenheimer, M.M., Banka, V.S., Fooshee, C.M., Hermann, G.A., and Helfant, R.H. Comparison of wall motion and regional ejection fraction at rest and during isometric exercise: concise communication. *J Nucl Med, 20*:724–732, 1979.

Bolstad, A., and Ersland, A. Energy metabolism in different human skeletal muscles during voluntary isometric contractions. *Eur J Appl Physiol, 38*:171–179, 1978.

Bowers, L. Effects of autosuggested muscle contraction on muscular strength and size. *Res Q, 37*:302–312, 1966.

Brown, G.L., and Burns, B.D. Fatigue and neuromuscular block in mammalian skeletal muscle. *Proc R Soc Lund* [Biol], 136:182, 1949.

Bruce, R., Gey, G.O., Cooper, M.N., Fisher, L.D., and Peterson, D.R. Seattle heart watch. Initial clinical, circulatory and electrocardiographic responses to maximal exercise. *Am J Cardiol, 33*:459–468, 1968.

Buchthal, F., Guld, C., and Rosenfalck, P. Action potential parameters in normal human muscle and their dependence on physical variables. *Acta Physiol Scand, 32*:200–229, 1954.

―――― Propagation velocity in electrically activated muscle fibres in man. *Acta Physiol Scand, 34*:75–89, 1955.

Buck, J.A., Amundsen, L., and Nielsen, D.H. Systolic blood pressure responses during isometric contractions of large and small muscle groups. *Med Sci Sports, 12*(3):145–147, 1980.

Buller, A.J., Eccles, J.C., and Eccles, R.M. Interactions between motor-neurons and muscle in respect to the characteristic speeds of their responses. *J Physiol, 150*:417, 1960.

Buller, A.J., and Lewis, D.M. The rate of tension in isometric contractions of mammalian fast and slow muscles. *J Physiol, 169*:29, 1966.

―――― Further observations on the differentiation of skeletal muscles in the kitten hind limb. *J Physiol, 176*:355–370, 1965.

―――― The rate of tension development in isometric tetanic contractions of mammalian fast and slow skeletal muscle. *J Physiol, 176*:337–354, 1965.

Buller, A.J., Mommaerts, W.M., and Seraydarian, K. Enzymic properties of myosin in fast and slow-twitch muscles of the cat following cross-innervation. *J Physiol, 205*:581-597, 1969.

―――― Neural control of myofibrillar ATPase activity in rat skeletal muscle. *Nature [New Biology], 31*:233, 1971.

Buller A.J., Ranatunga, K.W., and Smith, J.M. The influence of temperature on the contractile characteristics of mammalian fast and slow twitch skeletal muscles. *J Physiol, 196*:82, 1963.

Burke, R., Levine, N., and Zajac, F. Mammalian motor units: Physiological-histochemical correlation in three types in cat gastrocnemius. *Science, 176*:709–712, 1965.

Buskirk, E.R., Thompson, R.H., and Whelon, G.D. *Temperature — Its Measurement and Control in Science and Industry.* New York: Reinhold Publishing Co., 1963.

Byrd, R.J., and Hills, W.L. Strength, endurance, and blood flow responses to isometric training. *Res Q, 42*(4):357–361, 1972.

Caldwell, L.S. The load-endurance relationship for a static manual response. *Hum Factors, 6*:71–77, 1964.

Carlson, K., Alston, W., and Feldman, D. Electromyographic study of aging in skeletal muscle. *Am. J. Phys Med., 43*(4):141–145, 1964.

Carroll, D., and Rhys-Davies, L. Heart rate changes with exercise and voluntary heart rate acceleration. *Biol Psychol., 8*:241–252, 1979.

Cenkovich, F.S., and Gersten, J.W. Fourier analysis of the normal human electromyogram. *Am. J. Phys Med., 42*:192–204, 1963.

Chrysant, S.G. Hemodynamic effects of isometric exercise in normotensive hypertensive subjects hypertension. *Angiology, 29*(5):379–385, 1978.

Clamann, P.H. Activity of single motor units during isometric tension. *Neurology, 20*:254–260, 1970.

Clamann, P.H., and Borecker, K.T. Relations between force and fatiguability of red and pale muscles in man. *Am J Phys Med, 58*:70-85, 1979.

Clarke, R.S.J., Hellon, R.F., and Lind, A.R. The duration of sustained contractions of the human forearm at different muscle temperatures. *J Physiol, 143*:454–473, 1958.

Clement, D.L., Pelletier, C.L., and Shepard, J.T. Role of muscular contraction in the reflex vascular responses to stimulation of muscle afferents in the dog. *Circ Res., 33*:386–392, 1973.

Close, R.I. Dynamic properties of fast and slow skeletal muscles of the rat during development. *J Physiol, 176*:74–95, 1964.

——— Dynamic properties of mammalian skeletal muscles. *Physiol. Rev., 52*:129–197, 1972.

——— The relations between sarcomere length and characteristics of isometric twitch contractions of frog sartorius muscle. *J Physiol, 220*:745–762, 1972.

Close, R.I., and Hoh, J.F.Y. Influence of temperature on isometric contraction of rat skeletal muscles. *Nature, 217*:1178–1180, 1968.

Cobb, S., and Forbes, A. Electromyographic study of muscle fatigue in men. *Am J Physiol, 65*:234–251, 1923.

Coleman, E.A. Effect of unilateral isometric and isotonic contractions on the strength of the contralateral limb. *Res Q., 40*:490–495, 1969.

Cooley, J., and Tukey, J.W. An algorithm for the machine calculation of complex Fourier series. *Math Computations, 19*:297–301, 1965.

Coote, J.H., Hilton, S.M., and Perez-Gonzalez, J.F. The reflex nature of the pressor response to muscular isometric exercise. *J Physiol, 215*:789–804, 1971.

Corbett, J.S., Frankel, H.L., and Harris, P.J. Cardiovascular changes associated with skeletal muscle spasm in tetraplegic men. *J Physiol, 215*:381–387, 1970.

Cotton, D. Relationship of the duration of sustained voluntary isometric contraction to changes in endurance and strength. *Res Quart, 38*:366–374, 1970.

Cotton, D.J., and Bonnel, L. Investigation of the T5 cable tensionometer grip attachment for measuring strength of college women. *Res Quart, 40*:848–850, 1969.

Corr, P.B. Effect of autonomic neural influence on the cardiovascular changes induced by coronary occlusion. *Am Heart J, 89*(6):766–774, 1975.

Corr, P.B., and Gillis, R.A. Role of the vagus nerves in the cardiovascular changes induced by coronary occlusion. *Circulation, 49*:86–97, 1974.

Crawford, M.H., White, D.H., and Amon, K.W. Echocardiographic evaluation of left ventricular size and performance during handgrip and supine and upright bicycle exercise. *Circulation, 59*(6):1188–1196, 1979.

Crayton, S.C., Aung-Din, R., Fixler, D.E., and Mitchell, J.H. Distribution of cardiac output during induced isometric exercise in dogs. *Am J Physiol, 236*(2):H218–H224, 1979, or *Am J Physiol: Heart Circ Physiol, 5*(2):H218–H224, 1979.

Cullingham, P.J., Lind, A.R., and Morton, R.J. The maximal isometric tetanic tensions developed by mammalian muscle, *in situ* at different temperatures. *Q J Exp Physiol, 45*:142–151, 1965.

Daniels, R. Jr., and Baker, P.T. Relation between body fat and shivering in air at 15° C. *J Appl Physiol, 16*:421–426, 1961.

DeLorme, T.L., and Watkins, A.L. *Progressive Resistance Exercise.* New York: Appleton Century Inc. 1951.

Denny-Brown, D.E. The histological features of striped muscle in relation to its functional activity. *Proc R Soc,* 104:371–410, 1926.

———— On the nature of postural reflexes. *Proc R Soc. 104*:252–301, 1929.

DeVries, H.A. Efficiency of electrical activity as a measure of the functional state of muscle tissue. *Am J Phys Med, 47*:10–22, 1968.

———— Method for evaluation of muscle fatigue and endurance from electromyographic fatigue curves. *Am J Phys Med, 47*(3):125–135, 1968.

———— Method for evaluation of muscle fatigue and endurance from electromyographic curves. *Am J Phys Med, 47*:125–135, 1968.

DeVries, H.A., and Adams, G.M. Total muscle mass activation *vs.* relative loading of individual muscle as determinents of isometric response in older men. *Med Sci Sports, 4*:146–154, 1972.

Dickinson, S. The efficiency of bicycle pedalling, as affected by speed and load. *J Physiol,* 66: 242–255, 1929.

Dietz, H., and Volker, W. Analysis of the electrical muscle activity during maximal contraction and the influence of ischaemia. *J Neurol Sci.* 37: 187–197, 1978.

Donald, K.W., et al. Cardiovascular responses to static contractions. *Circ Res* 20: 115–130, 1967.

Drahota, A., and Guttman, E. Long term influence of the nervous system on some metabolic differences in muscles of different function. *Physiol Bohemoslov,* 12: 339, 1963.

Dubowitz, V., and Brooke, M.H. *Muscle Biopsy: A Modern Approach.* Philadelphia, Saunders, 1974.

Duling, B.R., and Pittman, R.N. Oxygen tension: dependent or independent blood flow? *Fed Proc, 134*:2012, 1975.

Dusser de Barenne, J.G., and Burger, G.C. Untersuchungen über den Gaswechsel des Menschen bei statischer Arbeit. *Pfluger Arch Ges Physiol, 218*:239–247, 1928.

Eason, R.G. Electromyographic study of local and generalized muscular impairment. *J Appl Physiol,* 15(3): 479–482, 1960.

Edstrom, L., and Nystrom B. Histochemical types of fibers and fiber size in human skeletal muscle. *ACTA Physiol Scand, 45*:257–269, 1969.

Edwards, R.H.T., and Lippold, O.C.J. The relation between force and integrated electrical activity in fatigued muscle. *J Physiol, 132*:677–681, 1956.

Edwards, R.H.T. Physiological analysis of skeletal muscle weakness and fatigue. *Clin Sci Mol Med, 54*:463–470, 1978.

Edwards, R.H.T., Harris, R.C., Hultman, E., Kaizer, L., Koh, D., and Nordesjo, L. Energy metabolism during isometric exercise at different temperature of M. Quadriceps Femoris in man. *ACTA Physiol Scand, 80*:17A–18A, 1975.

—— Effect of temperature on muscle energy metabolism and endurance during successive isometric contractions, sustained to fatigue, of the quadriceps muscle in man. *J Physiol, 220*:335–352, 1972.

Edwards, R.H.T., Harris, R.C., Hultman, E., and Nordesjo, L.O. Phosphagen utilization and resynthesis in successive isometric contractions, sustained to fatigue, of the quadriceps muscle in man. *J Physiol, 244*:40–41, 1972.

Edwards, R.H.T., Hill, D.K., and Jones, D.A. Heat production and chemical changes during isometric contractions of the human quadriceps muscles. *J Physiol, 251*:303–315, 1975.

—— Metabolic changes associated with the slowing and relaxation in fatigued mouse muscle. *J Physiol, 251*:287–301, 1975.

Edwards, R.H.T., Hill, D.K., Jones, D.A., and Merton, P.A. Fatigue of long duration in human skeletal muscle after exercise. *J Physiol, 272*:769–778, 1977.

Edwards, R.H.T., Hill, D.K., and McDonnell, M. Myothermal and intramuscular pressure measurements during isometric contractions of the human quadriceps muscle. *J Physiol, 244*:58–59, 1972.

Elbel, E.R. The relationship between leg strength and other body measurements. *J Appl Physiol, 2*: 197–210, 1949.

Eriksson, E., and Haggmark, T. Comparison of isometric muscle training and electrical stimulation supplementing isometric muscle training in the recovery after major knee ligament surgery: a preliminary report. *Am J Sports Med, 7*(3):169–171, 1979.

Ewing, D.J., Irving, J.B., Kerr, F., and Kirby, B.J. Static exercise in unrelated systemic hypertension. *Br Heart J., 35*:413–421, 1973.

Fink, R., and Luttgau, H.C. An evaluation of the membrane constants and the potassium conductance in metabolically exhausted muscle fibres. *J Physiol, 263*:215–238, 1976.

Fiori, P. "Interrelationship Between Static and Dynamic Exercise." Master's Physiology thesis, Wright State University, 1980.

Fisher, M.L., Nutter, D.O., Jacobs, W., and Schlant, R.C. Hemodynamic evaluation of isometric exercise testing in cardiac patients. *Cardiology, 35*:422–432, 1973.

Fitch, C., Chevli, R., Petrofsky, J.S., and Kopp, S.J. Sustained isometric contraction in muscle depleted of phosphocreatine. *Life Sci, 23*:1285–1292, 1978.

Fitch, C., Jellinek, M., Fitts, R.H., Baldwin, K.M., and Holloszy, J.O. Phosphorylated o-guanidinopropionate as a substitute for phosphocreatine in rat muscle. *Am J Physiol, 228*(4):1123–1125, 1975.

Fitch, C., Jellinek, M., and Mueller, E.J. Experimental depletion of creatine and phosphocreatine from skeletal muscle. *J Biol Chem, 249*(4):1060–1063, 1974.

Fitts, R.H., Booth, F.W., Winder, W.W., and Holloszy, J.O. Skeletal muscle respiratory capacity, endurance and glycogen utilization. *Am J Physiol, 228*:1029–1033, 1975.

Fitts, R.H., Nagle, F.J., and Cassens, R.G. Characteristics of skeletal muscle fiber types in the miniature pig and the effect of training. *Can J Physiol Pharmacol, 51*:825–831, 1973.

Fixler, D.W., Laird, W., Browne, R., Fitzgerald, V., Wilson, S., and Vance, R. Response of hypertensive adolescents to dynamic and isometric exercise stress. *Pediatrics, 64*(5), 1979.

Folkow, B., and Halicka, H.D. A comparison between "red" and "white" muscle with respect to blood supply, capillary surface area and oxygen uptake during rest and exercise. *Micro Res, 1*:1–14, 1968.

Forrester, T., and Lind, A.R. Identification of adenosine triphosphate in human plasma in the concentration in the venous effluent of forearm muscles before, during, and after sustained contractions. *J Physiol, 204*:347–364, 1969.

Frauendorf, H., Gelbrich, W., Kramer, H., and Reimer, W. Einfluss von lokaler Erwärmung auf die Elektrische und das Oberflachen-EMG. *Eur J Appl Physiol, 33*:339–346, 1974.

Freund, H.J., Budingen, H.J., and Dietz, V. Activity of single motor units from human forearm muscles during voluntary isometric contractions. *J Neurophysiol, 38*:933–944, 1975.

Freund, P.R., Hobbs, S.F., and Rowell, L.B. Cardiovascular responses to muscle ischemia in man — dependency on muscle mass. *J Appl Physiol, 45*(5):762–767, 1978.

Freund, P.R., Rowell, L.B., Murphy, T.M., Hobbs, S.F., and Butler, S.H. Blockade of the pressor response to muscle ischemia by sensory nerve block in man. *Am J Physiol, 237*(4):433–439, 1979, or *Am J Physiol: Heart Circ Physiol, 6*(4):433–439, 1979.

Freyschuss, U. Cardiovascular adjustments to somatomotor activation. The elicitation of increments in heart rate, aortic pressure and venomotor tone with the initiation of muscle contraction. *Acta Physiol Scand., 343*:(Supplement 1), 1980.

Freyschoss, L. Elicitation of heart rate and blood pressure increase on muscle contraction. *J Appl Physiol, 28*(6):758–761, 1970.

Frisk-Holmberg, M., Essen, B., Fredriksson, M., and Strom, G. Skeletal muscle fibre type composition in relation to arterial blood pressure during dynamic and static exercise. *Clin Sci Mol Med, 56*:335–340, 1979.

Funderburk, C.F., Hipskind, S.G., Welton, R.F., and Lind, A.R. The development of and recovery from muscular fatigue induced by static effort at different tensions. *J Appl Physiol, 37*:392–401, 1974.

Bibliography

Fusfeld, R.D. A study of the differentiated electromyogram. *Electroencephalogr Clin Neurophysiol, 33*:511–515, 1972.

—— Analysis of electromyographic signals by measurement of wave duration. *Electroencephalogr Clin Neurophysiol, 30*:337–344, 1971.

Gaskell, W.H. On the changes of the bloodstream in muscles through stimulation of their nerves. *J Anat, 11*:360–371, 1877.

Gollnick, P.D., Armstrong, R.B., Saubert, C.W., Piehl, K., and Saltin, B. Enzyme activity and fiber composition in skeletal muscle of untrained and trained men. *J Appl Physiol, 33*:312–319, 1972.

Gollnick, P.D., and King, D.W. Effect of exercise and training on mitochondria of rat skeleton muscle. *Am J Physiol, 216*:1502, 1969.

Gollnick, P.D., Sjodin, B., Karlsson, J., Jansson, E., and Saltis, B. Human soleus muscle: a comparison of fiber composition and enzyme activities. *Europ J Physiol, 348*:247–255, 1974.

Gollnick, P.D., Struck, P.J., and Bogyo, P.T. Lactic dehydrogenase activities of rat heart and skeleton muscle after exercise and training. *J Appl Physiol, 22*:623, 1967.

Goodwin, G.M., McCloskey, D.I., and Mitchell, J.H. Cardiovascular and respiratory responses to changes in central command during isometric exercise at constant muscle tension. *J Physiol, 226*:173–190, 1972.

Greenleaf, J.E., Bernauer, E.M., Young, H.L., Morse, J.T., Staley, R.W., Juhos, L.T., and Van Beaumont, W. Fluid and electrolyte shifts during bed rest with isometric and isotonic exercise. *J Appl Physiol, 42*(1):59–66, 1977.

Grey, S.D., Carlsson, E., and Staub, N.C. Site of increased vascular resistance during isometric muscle contraction. *Am J Physiol, 213*(3):683–689, 1967.

Grimby, L., and Hannerz, J. Firing rate and recruitment order of toe extensor motor units in different modes of voluntary contraction. *J Physiol, 264*:865–879, 1977.

—— Recruitment order of motor units on voluntary contraction: changes induced by proprioceptive afferent activity. *J Neurol Neurosurg Psychiatry, 31*:565–573, 1968.

—— Disturbances in voluntary recruitment order of low and high frequency motor units on blockades of proprioceptive afferent activity. *Acta Physiol Scand, 96*:207–216, 1976.

Grimby, L., Hannerz, J., and Hedman, B. Contraction time and voluntary discharge properties of individual short toe extensor motor units in man. *J Physiol, 191*–201, 1979.

Grossman, W., McLaurin, L., Saltz, S., Paraskos, J., Dalen, J., and Dexter, L. Changes in the inotropic state of the left ventricle during isometric exercise. *Br Heart J, 35*:697–704, 1973.

Gutman, E., and Hanzlekova, V. *Age Changes of the Neuromuscular System*. Bristol, Scientechnica Ltd., 1972.

Guttman R. *Spinal Cord Injuries, Comprehensive Management and Research*. Oxford: Blackwell Scientific Publications, 1976.

Guyton. *Medical Physiology*, Philadelphia: Saunders & Co., 1980.

Guyton. D.L., Hambrecht, F.T. Theory and design of capacitor electrodes for chronic stimulation. *Med Biol Eng Comput, 12*:613–619, 1974.

Haddy, F.J., and Scott, J.B. Metabolic factors in peripheral circulatory regulation. *Fed Proc, 34*:2006–2014, 1975.

Hajek, I., Gutmann, E., and Syrovy, I. Changes of proteolytic activity in denervated and renervated muscle. *Physiol Bohemoslov, 12*:330–338, 1963.

Hajek, I., Gutmann, E., and Syrovy, I. Proteolytic activity in muscles of old animals. *Physiol Bohemoslov, 14*:481–486, 1965.

Hall, V.E., Mendoz, E., and Fitch, B. Reduction of strength of muscle contractions by the application of moist heat to the overlying skin. *Arch of Phys Med, 28*:493–499, 1947.

Hannerz, J., and Grimby, L. The afferent influence on the voluntary firing range of individual motor units in man. *Muscle and Nerve, 2*:414–422, 1979.

Hansen, J.W. Effect of dynamic training on isometric endurance of the elbow flexors. *Int A Angew Arbeit Physiol, 23*:367, 1967.

Helfant, R.H., deVilla, M.A., and Meister, S.G. Effect of sustained isometric handgrip exercise on left ventricular performance. *Circulation, 44*:982–993, 1971.

Hellebrandt, F.A., Parrish, A.M., and Houtz, S.J. Cross education. *Arch Phys Med Rehabil, 28*:76–85, 1947.

Hettinger, T. *Isometrisches Muskel-training*. Stuttgart, Georg Thieme Verlag, 1968.

Hettinger, T., and Müller, E.A. Muskelleistung und Muskel-Training. *Arbeitsphysiologie, 15*:111–126, 1953.

Heyward, V. Influence of static strength and intramuscular occlusion on submaximal static muscle endurance. *Res Quart, 46*:393–401, 1975.

Heyward, V., and McCreary, L. Analysis of the static strength and relative endurance of women athletes. *Res Q, 48*(4):703–710, 1977.

Hill, A.V. The pressure developed in muscle during contractions. *J Physiol, 107*:518–526, 1948.

Hnik, P., Hudlicka, O., Kuchera, J., and Payne, R. Activation of muscle afferents by nonproprioceptive stimuli. *Am J Physiol, 217*:1451–1458, 1969.

Hnik, P., Kriz, N., Vyskocil, F., Smiesko, V., Mejsnar, J., Ujec, E., and Holas, M. Word-induced potassium changes in muscle venous effluent blood measured by ion-specific electrodes. *Pflugers Arch, 338*:177–181, 1973.

Hobbs, S.F., Rowell, L., and Smith, O.A. Increased cardiovascular responses to static exercise after neuromuscular blockade in baboons. *The Physiologist, 23*:120, 1980.

Hoel, B.L., Lorentsen, E., and Lund-Larsen, P.G. *Acta Med Scand, 188*:491–495, 1970.

Holloszy, J.O., and Booth, F.W. Biomedical adaptations to endurance exercise in muscle. *Annu Rev Physiol, 38*:273–291, 1976.

Houston, J., Atkins, J., and Blomquist, G. Isometric exercise and the heart. *Clin Res, 18*:70–77, 1970.

Hume, L., and Reuben, S.R. The effects of exercise on the amplitude of the first heart sound in normal subjects. *Am Heart J, 95*(1):4–11, 1978.

Humphreys, P.W., and Lind, A.R. The blood flow through active and inactive muscles of the forearm during sustained handgrip contractions. *J Physiol, 166*:120–135, 1963.

Ikai, M., and Steinhaus, A.H. Some factors modifying the expression of human strength. *J Appl Physiol, 16*(1):157–163, 1961.

Inman, V.T., Ralston, H.J., Saunders, M.B., Feinstein, B., and Wright, E.W., Jr., Relation of human electromyogram to muscular tension. *Electroencephalography and Clinical Neurology, 4*:187–194, 1952.

Ismail, H.M., and Ranatunga, K.W. Isometric tension development in a human skeletal muscle in relation to its working range of movement: The length-tension relation of biceps brachii muscle. *Exp Neurol, 62*:595–604, 1978.

Jackson, D.H. Isometric exercise in the heart. *Ala J Med Sci, 7*:310–312, 1970.

Johnson, B.L., and Nelson, J.K. Effect of different motivational techniques during training and in testing upon strength performance. *Res Q, 38*:630, 1967.

Johnson, D.G., Hayward, J.S., Jacobs, T.P., Collins, M.L., Eckerson, J.D., and Williams, R.H. Plasma norepinephrine responses of man in cold water. *J Appl Physiol, 43*(2):216–220, 1977.

Johnson, M.A., Polgar, D., and Appleton, D. Data on the distribution of fiber types in thirty-six human muscles. *J Neurol Sci, 18*:111–129, 1973.

Johnson, P.C. Local regulatory mechanisms in the microcirculation. *Fed Proc, 34*:2005, 1975.

Jones, D.A., Bigland-Ritchie, B., and Edwards, R.H.T. Excitation frequency and muscle fatigue: mechanical responses during voluntary and stimulated contractions. *Exp Neurol, 64*:401–413, 1979.

Josenhans, W.C.T. The isometric exercise performance of men who are overweight. *Internationale Zeitschrift fuer angewandte Physiologie einschliesslich Arbeitsphysiologie, 19*:173–182, 1962.

Kaiser, E., and Peterson, I. Frequency analysis of muscle action potentials during tetanic contraction. *Electromyography, 3*:5–16, 1963.

Kalia, M., Senapati, J.M., Parida, B., and Panda, A. Reflex increase in ventilation by muscle receptors with nonmedullated fibres (C fibres). *J Appl Physiol, 32*:189–193, 1972.

Kao, F.F., and Ray, L.H. Respiratory and circulatory responses of anaesthetized dogs to induced muscular work. *Am J Physiol, 179*:249–254, 1954.

Karlsson, J., Funderburk, C.F., Essen, B., and Lind, A.R. Constituents of human muscle in isometric fatigue. *J Appl Physiol, 38*(2):208–211, 1975.

Karlsson, J., and Ollander, B. Muscle metabolites with exhaustive static exercise of different duration. *Acta Physiol Scand, 86*:309–314, 1972.

Kasser, R.J., and Lehr, R.P. Electromyographic frequency response of the biceps brachii in an isometric contraction to fatigue. *Electromyogr Clin Neurophysiol, 19*:175–181, 1979.

Kearney, J.T., Stull, G.A., and Kirkendall, D. Isometric grip-flexion fatigue in females under conditions of normal and occluded circulation. *Amer Corr Ther J*, 30(1):7–11, 1976.

Keatinge, W.R., and Evans, M. Effects of food, alcohol, and hyoscine on body temperature and reflex responses of men immersed in cold water. *Lancet*, 2:176, 1960.

Keys, A., and Brozek, J. Body fat in adult men. *Physiol Rev*, 33:245, 1953.

Kilbrom, A. Circulatory and ventilatory effects of combined static and dynamic activities. *Scand J Rehab Med*, 10(6):99–104, 1978.

Kilbrom, A., and Brundin, T. Circulatory effects of isometric muscle contractions performed separately and in combination with dynamic exercise. *Eur J Appl Physiol*, 36:7–17, 1976.

Kiveloff, B., and Huber, O. Brief maximal isometric exercise in hypertension. *J Am Geriatr Soc*, 19(11):1006–1012, 1971.

Kivowitz, C., Parmley, W.W., Donoso, R., Marcus, H., Ganz, W., and Swan, H.J.C. Effects of isometric exercise on cardiac performance: the grip test. *Circulation*, 44:994–1002, 1971.

Kjellmer, I. Studies on exercise hyperemia. *Acta Physiol Scand*, 64 (Suppl. 244):1, 1964.

Kogi, K., and Hakomada, T. Slowing of the surface electromyogram and muscle strength in muscle fatigue. Reports of the Physiology Lab, Institute of Science and Labour, 60:27–41, 1962.

Komi, P.V., and Viitasalo, J. Signal characteristics of the EMG at different levels of muscle tension. *Acta Physiol Scand*, 96:267–276, 1976.

Komi, P.V., Viitasalo, J.T., Rauramaa, R., and Vihko, V. Effect of isometric strength training on mechanical, electrical, and metabolic aspects of muscle function. *Eur J Appl Physiol*, 40:45–55, 1978.

Kopec, J., and Hausmanowa-Petrusewisz, I. Zastosowonie analizy harmonicznych do ocery electronmyogramu. *Acta Physiol Pol*, 17:713–725, 1966.

Kosarov, D., Rokotova, N.A., Shapkov, Y.T., and Anissimova, N.P. Firing frequency of single motor units upon voluntary control of the isometric tension in human muscles. *Acta Physiol Pharmacol Bul*, 5:3–10, 1979.

Krayenbuehl, H.P., Rutishauser, W., Schoenbeck, M., and Amende, I. Evaluation of left ventricular function from isovolumic pressure measurements during isometric exercise. *Am J Cardiol*, 29:323–330, 1973.

Kroll, W. Isometric fatigue curves under varied intertrial recuperation periods. *Res Q*, 39(1):106–115, 1968.

Krnjevic, K., and Miledi, R. Presynoptic failure of neuromuscular propagation in rats. *J Physiol*, 149:1–22, 1959.

Kumazawa, T., and Mizumura, K. Thin-fibre receptors responding to mechanical, chemical, and thermal stimulation in the skeletal muscle of the dog. *J Physiol*, 273:179–194, 1977.

Kuroda, E., Klissouras, V., and Milsum, J.H. Electrical and metabolic activities and fatigue in human isometric contraction. *J Appl Physiol, 29*(3):358–367, 1970.

Larsson, L., Grimby, G., and Karlsson, J. Muscle strength and speed of movement in relation to age and muscle morphology. *J Appl Physiol, 46*(3):451–456, 1979.

Larsson, L., and Karlsson, J. Isometric and dynamic endurance as a function of age and skeletal muscle characteristics. *Acta Physiol Scand, 104*:129–136, 1978.

Larsson, L., Linderholm, H., and Ringqvist, T. The effect of sustained and rhythmic contractions on the electromyogram (EMG). *Acta Physiol Scand, 65*:310–318, 1965.

Le Fever, R., and De Luca, C. "The Contribution of Individual Motor Units to the EMG Power Spectrum." Proceedings of the 29th ACEMB Meetings, 1976.

Leitner, L.M., and Dejours, P. Reflex increase in ventilation induced by vibrations applied to the triceps surae muscles in the cat. *Respir Physiol, 12*:199–204, 1971.

Levitt, E.E., and Brady, J.P. Muscular endurance under hypnosis and in the motivated waking state. *Int J Clin Exp Hypn, 12*:21, 1964.

Liley, A.W., and North K.A.K. An electrical investigation of effects of repetitive stimulation on mammalian neuromuscular junction. *J Physiol, 120*:509–526, 1953.

Lind, A.R. Muscle fatigue and recovery from fatigue induced by sustained contractions. *J Physiol, 147*:162–171, 1959.

Lind, A.R. and McNicol, G.W. Circulatory responses to sustained handgrip contractions performed during other exercise, both rhythmic and static. *J Physiol, 192*:595–604, 1967.

Lind, A.R., McNicol, G.W., Bruce, R.A., MacDonald, H.R., and Donald, K.W. The cardiovascular responses to sustained contractions of a patient with unilateral syringomyelia. *Clin Sci, 35*:45–53, 1968.

Lind, A.R., McNicol, G.W., and Donald, K.W. Circulatory adjustments to sustained (static) muscular activity. In Evang, K., and Andersen, K.L. (Eds): *Physical Activity in Health and Disease.* Baltimore, Williams and Wilkins, 1966, pp. 38–63.

Lind, A.R., and Petrofsky, J.S. Amplitude of the surface electromyograms during fatiguing isometric contractions. *Muscle and Nerve, 2*:257–324, 1979.

Lind, A.R., Taylor, S.H., Humphreys, P.W., Kennelly, B.M., and Donald, K.W. The circulatory effects of sustained voluntary muscle contraction. *Clin Sci, 27*:229–244, 1964.

Lind, A.R., Williams, C., and Petrofsky, J.S. A Physiological basis for establishing repetitive lifting in industry. *Ergonomics,* in press.

Lindhard, J. Untersuchungen über statische Muskelarbeit. *Scand Arch Physiol,* *40*:145–195, 1920.

Lindström, L., Kadefors, R., and Petersen, I. An electromyographic index for localized muscle fatigue. *J Appl Physiol, 43*(4):750–754, 1977.

Lindström, L., Magnusson, R., and Petersen, I. Muscular fatigue and action potential conducting velocity changes studied with frequency analysis of EMG signals. *Electromyography, 4*:341–353, 1970.

Lippold, O.C.J. The relation between integrated action potentials in a human muscle and its isometric tension. *J Physiol, 117*:492–499, 1952.

Lippold, O.C.J., Redfearn, J.W.T., and Vuco, J. The effect of sinusoidal stretching upon the activity of stretch receptors in voluntary muscle and their reflex responses. *J Physiol, 144,*:373–386, 1958.

———— The electromyography of fatigue. *Ergonomics, 3*:121–131, 1960.

Liu, C.T., Huggins, R.A., and Hoff, H.E. Mechanisms of intra-arterial K^+-induced cardiovascular respiratory responses. *Am J Physiol, 217*:969–973, 1969.

Lloyd, A.J., Voor, J.H., and Thieman, T.J. Subjective and electromyographic assessment of isometric muscle contractions. *Ergonomics, 13*(6):685–691, 1970.

Longhurst, J.C., Kelly, A., Gonyea, W., and Mitchell, J. Cardiovascular responses to static exercise in distance runners and weight lifters. *J of Appl Physiol, 49*:676–684, 1980.

Ludbrok, J., Faris, I.B., Jamieson, G.G., and Russell, W.J. Lack of effect of isometric handgrip exercise on the responses of the carotid sinus baroreceptor reflex in man. *Clin Sci Mol Med, 55*:189–194, 1978.

Lynn, P. Direct on-line estimation of muscle fiber conduction velocity by surface electromyography. *IEEE Trans Bio Eng, 26*:564–571, 1978.

McAllister, R.G., Jr. Effect of adrenergic receptor blockade on the responses to isometric handgrip: studies in normal and hypertensive subjects. *J Cardio Pharmacol, 1*:253–263, 1979.

McCloskey, D.I., and Mitchell, J.H. Reflex cardiovascular and respiratory responses originating in exercising muscle. *J Physiol, 224*:173–186, 1972.

McCloskey, D.I., and Streatfeild, K.A. Muscular reflex stimuli to the cardiovascular system during isometric contractions of muscle groups of different mass. *J Physiol, 250*:431–441, 1975.

Macdonald, H.R., Sapru, R.P., Taylor, S.H., and Donald, K.W. Effect of intravenous propranolol on the systems circulatory responses to sustained hand grip. *Am J Cardiol, 18*:333–344, 1966.

McGlynn, G.H. The relationship between maximum strength and endurance of individuals with different levels of strength. *Res Quart, 40*:529–535, 1969.

Mancia, G., Iannos, J., Jamieson, G.G., Lawrence, R.H., Sharman P.R., and Ludbrook, J. Effect of isometric handgrip exercise on the carotid sinus baroreceptor reflex in man. *Clin Sci Mol Med, 54*:33–37, 1967.

Marsden, D.D., Medows, J.C., and Merton, P. Isolated single motor units in human muscles and their rates of discharge during maximal voluntary effort. *J Physiol, 217*:12–13P, 1976.

Martens, R., and Sharkey, B.J. Relationship of phasic and static strength and endurance. *Res Q, 37*:435, 1966.

Martin, C.E., Shaver, J.A., Leon, D.F., Thompson, M.E., Reddy, P.S., and Leonard, J.J. Autonomic mechanisms in hemodynamic responses to isometric exercise. *J Clin Invest, 54*:104–115, 1974.

Maton, B. Motor unit differentiation and integrated surface EMG in voluntary isometric contraction. *Eur J Appl Physiol, 40*:150–159, 1976.

Matthews, O.A., Blomqvist, C.G., Cohen, L.S., and Mullins, C.B. *Circulation, 42*:111–131, 1970.

Mazzella, H. On the pressure developed by the contraction of striated muscle and its influence on muscular circulation. *Arch Internationales de Physiol, 42*:334–347, 1954.

Mense, M. Nervous outflow from skeletal muscle following chemical noxious stimulation. *J Physiol, 267*:75–88, 1977.

Merton, P.A. Voluntary strength and fatigue. *J Physiol, 123*:553–564, 1954.

Milner-Brown, H.S., and Stein, R.B. The relation between the surface electromyogram and muscular force. *J Physiol, 246*:549–569, 1975.

Merton, P.A. The properties of the human muscle servo. *Brain Research, 71*:475–478, 1974.

Mitchell, J. Muscle mass and the cardiovascular responses to static effort. *Circ Res,* in press.

Mitchell, J.H. Cardiovascular physiology of dynamic and static exercise. *Trans Assoc Life Ins Med Dir Am, 59*:147–153, 1976.

Mitchell, J.H., Reardon, W.C., McCloskey, D.I., and Wildenthal, K. Possible role of muscle receptors in the cardiovascular response to exercise. *Ann NY Acad Sci, 301*:232–242, 1981.

Mitchell, J.H., Reardon, W.C., and McCloskey, D.I. Reflex effects on circulation and respiration from contracting skeletal muscle. *Am J Physiol, 233*(3):374–378, 1977.

Mitchell, J.H., Schibye, B., Payne, F.C., and Saltin, B. Responses of arterial blood pressure to static exercise in relation to muscle mass, force development, and electromyographic activity. *Cir Res, 48*:70–75, 1981.

Mitchell, J.H., and Wildenthal, K. Static (isometric) exercise and the heart: physiological and clinical considerations. *Ann Rev Med, 25*:369–381, 1974.

Miyazawa, K., Haneda, T., Shirato, K., Honna, T., and Takishima, T. Effects of isometric handgrip exercise on coronary sinus blood in idiopathic cardiomyopathy. *Tohoku J Exp Med, 122*:1–8, 1977.

Miyazawa, K., Honna, T., Haneda, T., Arai, T., Nakajima, T., Miura, T., Kanazawa, M., and Onodera, S. Cineventriculographic Analysis of Left Ventricular Dynamics during Sustained Handgrip Exercise. *Tohoku J Exp Med, 130*:63–70, 1980.

Mohrman, E.E., Cant, J.R., and Sparks, H.B. Time course of vascular resistance and venous oxygen changes following brief tetanus of dog skeletal muscle. *Circ Res, 33*:316–323, 1973*b*.

Mohrman, E.E., and Sparks, H.V. Resistance and venous O₂ dynamics during sinusoidal exercise of dog skeletal muscle. *Circ Res, 33*:323–331, 1973*a*.

———— Myogenic hyperemia following brief tetanus of canine skeletal muscle. *Am J Physiol, 227*:531–537, 1974*a*.

———— Role of potassium ions in the vascular response to a brief tetanus. *Circ Res, 35*:384–391, 1974*b*.

Molbeck, S., and Johansen, S. Endurance time in static work during partial curarization. *J Appl Physiol, 27*:44, 1969.

Monod, H., and Scherrer, J. Capacite de travail staique d'une groupe musculaire synergique chez l'homme. *C R Soc Biol, 151*:1358–1369, 1967.

Monster, A.W. Firing rate behavior of human motor units during isometric voluntary contraction: relation to unit size. *Brain Res, 171*:349–354, 1979.

Moosa, A., and Brown, B.H. Quantitative electromyography: a new analogue technique for detecting changes in action potential duration. *J Neurol Neurosurg Psychiatry, 35*:216–220, 1972.

Morganroth, M.L., Mohrman, D.E., and Sparks, H.V. Prolonged vasodilation following fatiguing exercise of dog skeletal muscle. *Am J Physiol, 229*:38–47, 1975.

Moritani, T., and DeVries, H.A. Reexamination of the relationship between the surface integrated electromyogram (IEMG) and force of isometric contraction. *Am J Phys Med, 57*(6):263–277, 1978.

———— Neural factors versus hypertrophy in the time course of muscle strength gain. *Am J Phys Med, 58*(3):115–130, 1979.

Mortimer, J.T., Magnusson, R., and Petersen, I. Conduction velocity in ischemic muscle: effect on EMG frequency spectrum. *Am J Physiol, 219*(5):1324–1329, 1970.

Mösseler, U., and Schlepper, M. Kreislaufforschungs, Z. *60*:1067–1073, 1971.

Muir, A.S., and Donald, K.W. *Proc R Soc, 63*:203–204, 1968.

Muller, E.A. Die physische Ermudung. *Handb Ges Arbeitsmedizin, 1*:405, 1961.

———— Influence of training and of inactivity on muscle strength. *Arch Phys Med Rehabil, 51*:440–461, 1970.

Muller, E.A., and Hettinger, T. Über Unterschiede der Trainingsgeschwindigkeit atrophierter und normaler Muskeln. *Arbeitsphysiol, 15*:223, 1953.

———— Muskelleistung und Muskeltraining. *Arbeitsphysiologie, 15*:111, 1953.

Muller, E.A., and Rohmert, W. Die Geschwindigkeit der Muskelkraft-Zunahme bei isometrischen Training. *Intern Z Angew Physiol, 19*:403, 1963.

Mullins, C.B., Leshin, S.J., Mierzwiak, D.S., Matthews, O.A., and Blomqvist, C.G. Sustained forearm contraction (handgrip) as a stress test for evaluation of left ventricular function. *Clin Res, 18*:322, 1970.

Murray, M.P., Gardner, G.M., Mollinger, L.A., and Sepic, S.B. Strength of isometric and isokinetic contractions: knee muscles of men aged 20-86. *Phys Ther, 60*(4):412–419, 1980.

Myhre, K., and Anderson, K.L. Respiratory responses to static muscular work. *Resp Physiol, 12*:77–89, 1971.

Nudel, D.B., Gootman, N., Brunson, S., Stenzler, A., Shenker, I.R., and Gauthier, B.G. Exercise performance of hypertensive adolescents. *Pediatrics, 65*(6), 1073–1078, 1980.

Nyberg, G., Vedin, A., and Wilhelmsson, C. Effects of labetalol and propranolol on blood pressure at rest and during isometric and dynamic exercise. *Eur J Clin Pharmacol, 16*:299–303, 1979.

Ochs, R.M., Smith, J.L., and Edgerton, V.R. Fatigue characteristics of human gastrocnemius and soleus muscles. *Electromyogr Clin Neurophysiol, 17*:297–306, 1977.

Olson, C.B., Carpenter, D.O., and Henneman, E. Orderly recruitment of muscle action potentials. *Arch Neurol, 19*:591–597, 1968.

Ordway, G.A., and Wekstein, D.R. The effect of age on selected cardiovascular responses to static (isometric) exercise. *Soc for Exp Biol and Med, 161*:189–192, 1979.

Ortengren, R. A filter bank analyser with simultaneous readout for the evaluation of dynamic myoelectric signal power spectra. *Med Biol Eng Comput, (July)*:561–569, 1975.

Parfrey, P.S., Wright, P., and Ledingham, J.M. Effect of isometric exercise on the renal excretion of sodium and potassium in mild hypertension. *Clin Sci, 57*:317–320, 1979.

Paulsen, W.J., Boughner, D.R., Friesen, A., and Persaud, J.A. Ventricular response to isometric and isotonic exercise: echocardiographic assessment. *Br Heart J, 42*:521–527, 1979.

Pearce, K.I., and Shaw, J.C. Activity measurement using the integrating and crossover counters. *Med Electron Biol Eng, 3*:189–198, 1965.

Perez, J.E., Cintron, G., Gonzalez, M., Hernandez, E., Linares, E., and Aranda, J. Hemodynamic response to isometric handgrip in acute myocardial infarction. *Chest, 77*:194–197, 1980.

Pernow, B., and Saltin, B. *Muscle Meta Exer*, New York: Plenum, 1971.

Petersen, F.B., Graudal, H., Hansen, J.W., and Hvid, N. The effect of varying the number of muscle contractions on dynamic muscle training. *Intern Z Angew Physiol, 18*:468, 1961.

Petrofsky, J.S. Computer analysis of the surface EMG during isometric exercise. *Comput Biol Med, 10*:83–95, 1980.

——— Control of the recruitment and firing frequencies of motor units in electrically stimulated muscles in the cat. *Med Biol Eng Comput, 16*:302–308, 1978.

——— Digital analogue hybrid 3 channel sequential stimulator. *Med Biol Eng Comput, 17*:421–424, 1979.

——— Filter bank analyzer for the automatic analysis of the EMG. *Med Biol Eng Comput 18*:585–590, 1980.

——— Frequency and ampitude analysis of the EMG during exercise on the bicycle ergometer. *Eur J Appl Physiol, 41*:1–15, 1979.

———— The influence of recruitment order and temperature on tension development and fatigability of mammalian skeletal muscles; with special reference to motor unit fatigue. *Eur J Appl Physiol*, in press.

———— *In vivo* measurement of brain blood flow in the cat. *IEEE Trans Biomed Eng, BME-26*:441–444, 1979.

———— Motor unit recruitment patterns during submaximal isometric contractions. Submitted to *J Appl Physiol*, 1981c.

———— A portable digital force dynamometer. *IEEE NAECON Record*, 570–574 pp., 1981.

———— Quantification of fatigue during successive isometric contractions. *Proc Aerospace Med Assoc*, 215–216, 1980.

———— Quantification through the surface EMG of muscle fatique and recovery during successive isometric contractions. *Aviat Space Env Med, 52*:545-550, 1981.

———— Sequential motor unit stimulation through peripheral motor nerves. *Med Biol Eng Comput, 17*:87–93, 1979.

Petrofsky, J.S., Betts, W., Lind, A.R. Quantification of the surface EMG. *Fed Proc, 36*:1194, 1977.

Petrofsky, J.S., Burse, R., and Lind, A.R. The effect of deep muscle temperature on the cardiovascular responses of man to static effort. *Eur J Appl Physiol*, in press.

———— Comparison of physiological responses of women and men to isometric exercise. *J Appl Physiol, 38*:863–868, 1975.

Petrofsky, J.S., Dahms, T.E., and Lind, A.R. Power spectrum analysis of the EMG during static exercise. *Physiologist, 18*:350, 1975.

Petrofsky, J.S., and Fitch, C. Contractile characteristics of skeletal muscle depleted of phosphocreatinine. *Eur J Physiol, 384*:123–129, 1980.

Petrofsky, J.S., Guard, A., and Lind, A.R. The influence of muscle temperature on the contractile characteristics of fast and slow muscle in the cat. *Physiologist, 21*:91, 1978.

Petrofsky, J.S., Guard, A., and Phillips, C.A. The effect of muscle fatigue on the isometric contractile characteristics of fast and slow twitch skeletal muscle in the cat. *Life Sci, 24*:2285–2292, 1979.

Petrofsky, J.S., LaDonne, D., Reinhart, J.S., and Lind, A.R. The influence of the menstrual cycle on blood flow through muscle during isometric contractions. *Ohio J Science*, in press.

———— Isometric strength and endurance during the menstrual cycle in healthy young women. *Eur J Appl Physiol, 35*:1–10, 1976.

Petrofsky, J.S., and Lind, A.R. Aging, isometric strength and endurance, and the cardiovascular responses to static effort. *J Appl Physiol, 38*:91–95, 1975.

———— The blood pressure response during isometric exercise in fast and slow twitch skeletal muscle in the cat. *Eur J Appl Physiol, 44*:223–230, 1980.

———— Blood pressure response in fast and slow muscle in the cat, submitted to *Life Sci*, 1979.

——— Comparison of metabolic and ventilatory responses of men to various lifting tasks and bicycle ergometry. *J Appl Physiol, 45*:60–63, 1980.

——— Frequency analysis of the surface EMG during sustained isometric exercise. *Eur J Appl Physiol, 43*:173–182, 1980.

——— The influence of temperature on the amplitude and frequency components of the EMG during brief and sustained isometric contractions. *Eur J Appl Physiol, 44*:1980.

——— The influence of temperature on the isometric characteristics of fast and slow muscle in the cat. *Eur J Physiol, 389*:149–154, 1981.

——— The insulative power of body fat on deep muscle temperature and isometric endurance. *J Appl Physiol, 39*:639–642, 1969.

——— Isometric endurance in fast and slow muscles in the cat. *Am J Physiol, 236*:185–191, 1979.

——— Isometric strength, endurance, and the blood pressure and heart rate responses during isometric exercise in healthy men and women, with special reference to age and body fat content. *Pflugers Arch, 360*:49–61, 1975.

——— Metabolic, cardiovascular and respiratory factors in the development of fatigue in lifting tasks. *J Appl. Physiol, 45*:270–274, 1978.

——— The relationship of body fat content to deep muscle temperature and isometric endurance in man. *Clin Sci Mol Med, 48*:405–412, 1975.

Petrofsky, J.S., and Phillips, C.A. Constant velocity contractions in skeletal muscle of the cat. *Med Biol Eng Comput, 17*:583–592, 1979.

——— Determination of the contractile characteristics of the motor units in skeletal muscle through twitch characteristics. *Med Biol Eng Comput, 17*:525–533, 1979.

——— The effect of elbow angle on isometric strength and endurance of the biceps in men and women. *J Hum Ergol*, in press.

——— The impact of recruitment order on electrode design for neural prothesis. *Am J Phys Med*, in press.

——— The influence of recruitment order and fibre composition on the force-velocity relationship and fatigability of skeletal muscle in the cat. *Med Biol Eng Comput, 18*:381–390, 1980.

——— Interrelationship between muscle fatigue, muscle temperature, blood flow and the surface EMG. *IEEE NAECON Record*, 520–527, 1980.

——— Microprocessor stimulation of paralyzed muscle. *IEEE NAECON Record*, 198–210, 1979.

——— The relationship between body fat and the recovery of strength and endurance following isometric exercise. *Ergonomics, 24*:215–222, 1981.

——— The relationship between temperature and muscle length on the force-velocity relationship. *J Biomech, 14*:297–306, 1981.

Petrofsky, J.S., Phillips, C.A., and Lind, A.R. Interrelationships between recruitment order, muscle temperature, and endurance for static exercise and the blood pressure response in the cat. *Circ Res, 48*:I-32–I-36, 1981.

Petrofsky, J.S., Phillips, C.A., Lind, A.R., Sawka, D., Hanpeter, D., and Stafford, D. Muscle fiber recruitment and the blood pressure response to isometric exercise. *J Appl Physiol, 50*:32–37, 1981.

Petrofsky, J.S., Phillips, C.A., Sawka, M., Hanpeter, D., and Stafford, D. Blood flow and metabolic products during fatiguing isometric contractions in fast and slow skeletal muscles in the cat. *J Appl Physiol, 50*:493–502, 1981.

Petrofsky, J.S., Phillips, C.A., Sawka, M., Hanpeter, D. and Weber, C. Mechanical, electrical, and biochemical correlates of isometric fatigue in the cat. *Advances in Physiol, 18*:229–236, 1980.

Petrofsky, J.S., Rochelle, R.H., Rinehart, J.S., Burse, R.L., and Lind, A.R. The assessment of static component in rhythmic exercise. *Eur J Appl Physiol, 34*:55–63, 1975.

Petrofsky, J.S., Weber, C., and Phillips, C.A. Electrical and mechanical correlates of fatigue in skeletal muscle. *The Physiologist, 22*:101, 1979.

———— Mechanical and electrical correlates of isometric muscle fatigue in skeletal muscle in the cat. *Europ J Physiol, 387*:33–38, 1980.

Petrofsky, J.S., Williams, C.A., Kamen, G., and Lind, A.R. The effect of handgrip span on isometric performance. *Ergonomics*, in press.

Pette, D., Ramirez, B., Muller, W., et al. Influence of intermittent long-term stimulation on contractile, histochemical and metabolic properties of fibre populations in fast and slow rabbit muscles. *Pfluegers Arch, 361*:1–7, 1975.

Pette, D., Smith, M.E., Staudte, H.W., et al. Effects of long-term electrical stimulation on some contractile and metabolic characteristics of fast rabbit muscles. *Pfluegers Arch, 338*:257–272, 1973.

Pette, D., Staudte, H.W., and Vrbova, G. Physiological and biochemical changes induced by long-term stimulation of fast muscle. *Naturwissenschaften, 59*:469–470, 1972.

Piper, H. *Elektrophysiologie menschlicher Muskeln*, Berlin: Springer, 1912, p. 126.

Quinones, M.A., Gaasch, W.H., and Wasser, E. An analysis of the left-ventricular response to isometric exercise. *Am Heart J, 88*:29–36, 1974.

Rack, P.M.H., and Westbury, D.R. The effects of length and stimulus rate on tension in the isometric cat soleus muscle. *J Physiol, 204*:443–460, 1969.

Ranson, S.W., and Davenport, H.K. Sensory unmyelinated fibers in the spinal nerves. *Am J Anat, 48*:331–353, 1931.

Reid, C. The mechanism of voluntary muscle fatigue. *Quart J Exp Physiol, 19*:17–31, 1928.

Reis, D.J., and Wooten, G.F. The relationship of blood flow to myoglobin, capillary density, and twitch characteristics in red and white skeletal muscle in cat. *J Physiol, 210*:121–135, 1970.

Reuben, S.R., Gale, E.V., and Blake, P. The effects of α and β-adrenergic receptor blockers on the pressure responses to isometric exercise in hypertensive patients. *Br J Clin Pharmacol, 8*:365–368, 1979.

Robson, D.H., and Fluck, D.C. Effect of isometric exercise on catecholamines in the coronary circulation. *Europ J Appl Physiol, 38*:291–295, 1977.

Rodbard, S., and Pragay, E.B. Contraction frequency, blood supply, and muscle pain. *J Appl Physiol, 24*:142–145, 1968.

Roddie, I.C., and Shepherd, J.T. Nervous control of the circulation in skeletal muscle. *Br Med Bull, 19*(2):115–119, 1967.

Rohmert, W. Physiologische Grundlagen der Erholungszeitbestimmung. *Zbl Arbeit Wiss, 19*:1, 1965.

——— Rechts-links Vergleich bei isometrischem Armmuskeltraining mit verschiedenem Trainingsreiz bei achtjährigen Kindern. *Int Z angew Physiol, 26*:363, 1968.

——— Untersuchung statischer Haltearbeiten in achtstundigen Arbeitsversuchen. *Int Z angew Physiol, 19*:35, 1961.

——— Ermittlung von Erholungspausen für statische Arbeit des Menschen. *Int Z angew Physiol, 18*:123–128, 1960.

Rohter, F.D., Rochelle, R.H., and Hyman, C.J. Exercise blood flow changes in the human forearm during physical training. *J Appl Physiol, 18*:789–93, 1963.

Rowell, L.B., Hermansen, L., and Blackmon J.R. Human cardiovascular and respiratory responses to graded muscle ischemia. *J Appl Physiol, 41*(5):693–701, 1976.

Royce, J. Isometric fatigue curves in human muscle with normal and occluded circulation. *Res Q, 29*(2):204–212, 1957.

Rozier, C.K., Elder, J.D., and Brown, M. Prevention of atrophy by isometric exercises of a casted leg. *J Sports Med Phys Fitness, 19*(2):191–194, 1979.

Saltin, B., Blomqvist, B., Mitchell, J.H., Johnson, R.L., Wildenthal, K., and Chapman, C.B. Response to submaximal and maximal exercise after bed rest and training. *Circulation, 38*:(Suppl. 7), 1968.

Saltin, B., Mitchell, J.H., Schibye, B., and Payne, F.C. Role of muscle mass in the cardiovascular response to isometric contractions. *Acta Physiol Scand, 102*:79–80, 1978.

Sanchez, J., Monod, H., and Chabaud, F. Effects of dynamic static and combined work on heart rate and oxygen consumption. *Ergonomics, 22*:935–943, 1979.

Sano, T., Motomiya, T., and Yamazaki, H. Platelet release reaction in vivo in patients with ischaemic heart disease after isometric exercise and its prevention with dipyridamole. *Thromb Haemost, 42*:1589–1597, 1977.

Savin, W.M., Alderman, E.L., Haskell, W.L., Schroeder, J.S., Ingels, N.B., Daughters, G.T., and Stinson, E.B. Left ventricular response to isometric exercise in patients with denervated and innervated hearts. *Circulation, 61*(5):897–901, 1980.

Sawka, M., Petrofsky, J.S., and Phillips, C.A. Energy cost of isometric contractions in fast and slow-twitch skeletal muscle. *Europ J Physiol, 390*:164–168, 1981.

Serfass, R.C., Stull, G.A., Ben-Sira, D., and Kearney, J.T. Effects of circulatory occulusion on submaximal isometric endurance. *Am Corr Ther J, 33*:147–154, 1979.

Schmalboruch, H., and ·Kamienecka, Z. Fiber types in the human brachial biceps muscle. *Exp Neurol, 44*:313–328, 1974.

Shaver, L.G. Relation of maximum isometric strength and relative isotonic endurance of the elbow flexors of athletes. *Res Q, 43*(1):82–88, 1972.

Shepard, J., and Vanhoutte. *Human Cardiovascular System.* New York, Raven Press, 1979.

Siegel, W., Gilbert, C.A., Nutter, D.O., Schlant, R.C., and Hurst, J.W. *Am J Cardiol, 30*:48–54, 1972.

——— L'adaption au travail physique. *Travail Humain, 4*:129, 1936.

Simonson, E., *Physiology of Work Capacity and Fatigue.* Springfield, Thomas, 1971.

——— Weitere Beitraege zur Physiologie der Atmung und Übung. *Pflueger Arch Ges Physiol, 215*:752, 1927*b*.

——— Zur Physiologie des Energieumsatze beim Menschen. III. Weitere Beitrage zur Physiologie der Erholung bei koerperlicher Arbeit. *Pflueger Arch Ges Physiol, 215*:716, 1927*a*.

Simonson, E., and Hebestreit, H. Zum Verhalten des Wirkungsgrades bei korperlicher Arbeit. VII. Zur Physiologie des Energieumsatzes. *Pflueger Arch Ges Physiol, 225*:498, 1930.

Stafford, D., and Petrofsky, J.S. The relationship between fatiguing and non-fatiguing isometric contractions. Submitted to *J Appl Physiol, 51*:399–404, 1981.

Start, K.B., and Graham, J.S. The relation between relative and absolute endurance of an isolated muscle group. *Res Q, 35*:193, 1964.

Staunton, H.P., Taylor, S.H., and Donald, K.W. The effect of vascular occlusion on the pressor response to static muscular work. *Clin Sci, 27*:283–291, 1964.

Stephens, J.A., and Taylor, A. An analysis of muscle fatigue mechanisms in man. *J Physiol, 220*:1–18, 1972.

——— Fatigue of maintained voluntary muscle contraction in man. *J Physiol, 220*:1–18, 1972.

Stillwell, D.M., McLarren, G.L., and Gersten, J.W. Atrophy of quadriceps muscle due to immobilization of lower extremity. *Arch Phys Med Rehabil, 48*:289–295, 1967.

Stulen, F.B., and DeLuca, C.J. *A Non-Invasive Device for Monitoring Metabolic Correlates of Myoelectric Signals.* Paper read at 31st ACEMB, 21-25, October 1978, Marriott Hotel, Atlanta, Georgia.

Sylvest, O., and Hvid, N. Pressure measurements in human striated muscles during contraction. *Acta Rheumatica Scandinavica, 5*:216, 1959.

Tibes, U. Reflex inputs to the cardiovascular and respiratory centers from dynamic working canine muscles: some evidence for involvement of group III or IV nerve fibers. *Circ Res, 41*:332–341, 1977.

Tornvall, G. Assessment of physical capabilities with special reference to the evaluation of maximal voluntary isometric muscle strength and maximal working capacity. An experimental study on civilian and military subject groups. *Acta Physiol Scand, 58* (Suppl. 201):1, 1963.

Tuttle, W.W., and Horvath, S.M. Comparison of effects of static and dynamic work on blood pressure and heart rate. *J Appl Physiol, 10*:294–296, 1957.

Vanderhoff, E.R., Imig, C.J., and Hines, H.M. Effect of muscle strength and endurance development on blood flow. *J Appl Physiol, 16*:873–877, 1961.

Viitasalo, J.H.T., and Komi, P.V. Signal characteristics of EMG during fatigue. *Eur J Appl Physiol, 37*:111–121, 1977.

Vrbóva, G. The effect of motoneurons activity on the speed of contraction of striate muscle. *J Physiol, 169*:513–526, 1963.

Wildenthal, K., Mierzwiak, D.S., Skinner, N.S., and Mitchell, J.H. Potassium-induced cardiovascular and ventilatory reflexes from the dog hindlimb. *Am J Physiol, 215*:542–548, 1968.

Wiley, R.L., and Lind, A.R. Respiratory responses to simultaneous static and rhythmic exercises in humans. *Clin Sci Mol Med, 49*:427–432, 1975.

———— Respiratory responses to sustained static muscle contractions in man. *Fed Proc, 29*(2):265, 1970.

———— Respiratory responses to sustained static muscular contractions in humans. *Clin Sci, 40*:221–234, 1971.

Williams C.A., Petrofsky, J.S., and Lind, A.R. Cardiovascular responses to lifting in women. Submitted to *Eur J Appl Physiol*, 1981.

Wilmore, J.H. Individual exercise prescription. *Am J Cardiol, 33*:757–759, 1974.

Yoo, J.H.K., Herring, J.M., and Yu, J. Power spectral changes of the vastus medialis electromyogram for graded isometric torques (1). *Electromyogr Clin Neurophysiol, 19*:183–197, 1979.

Zajac, F. Recruitment and rate modulation of motor units during locomotion. In Desmedt: *Progress in Clinical Neurophysiology*. Basel, Karger, 1978.

Zuniga, E.N., and Simmons, D.G. Non-linear relationship between averaged electromyograms potential and muscle tension in normal subjects. *Arch Phys Med Rehabil, 50*:264–272, 1969.

Zuntz, N., and Geppert, J. Über die Natur der normalen Atemreize und den Grad ihrer Wirkung. *Pfluegers Arch, 38*:337–345, 1888.

INDEX

fatigue
  ATP, 99
  ATPase activity, 102
  central, 104
  central nervous system, 106
  EMG, 56, 63, 107
  frequency of motor unit discharge, 106
  glycogen, 99
  hypnosis, 104
  lactic acid, 99, 100
  motor unit discharge, 106
  muscle temperature, 103
  muscle twitch, 103
  neuromuscular failure, 104
  posttetanic potentiation, 102
  recovery EMG, 63
  sustained maximal effort, 105
  velocity of shortening, 102
fatiguing isometric contractions, 69
frequency of discharge
  sustained contraction, 106

G
glycogen
  cat, 101
  man, 99

H
heart disease
  blood pressure, 125, 128
  cardiac output, 125
  coronary blood flow, 125
  role of vagal tone, 127
  stroke work, 126
heart rate
  aging, 85
  central component, 86
  dynamic exercise, 83
  mechanism, 85
  static exercise, 84
  tension, 86
hypertension, 129
hyperventilation, 89
hypnosis, 104

I
immobilization, 3
intramuscular pressure, 6, 9
isokinetics, 4

L
lactic acid
  cat, 101
  man, 99, 100
LVEDP, 125, 128, 129

M
motor unit action potential, 41
motor unit discharge
  fatigue, 106
muscle length
  EMG amplitude, 47
  strength, 11
muscle temperature
  EMG, 45
  fatigue, 103

N
neuromuscular junction
  fatigue, 104

P
potassium, 84

R
recovery
  effect of light exercise, 33
  effect of temperature, 31
  time course, 31
recruitment
  fast and slow muscle, 37, 38
  fatigue, 39
  frequency of discharge, 37, 39, 55
  pattern, 37, 39
  synchronization, 40, 41

S
sex differences
  blood pressure, 73
skin temperature
  EMG, 46
static component of dynamic work
  efficiency, 118
  endurance, 117, 120
strength
  hypnosis, 5
  motivation, 5, 13
  muscle length, 11
  relation to endurance, 14
  reliability, 11